CNA: A Person-Centered Approach Supplemental Manual

Table of Contents

Appendix A

Glossary of Terms

A

Abandonment: leaving a resident unattended

Abduction: away from the center (midline) of the body.

Abrasion: a scraping or rubbing off of the skin

Abuse: (verbal, physical or sexual abuse) "Abuse is the willful infliction of injury, unreasonable confinement, intimidation, or punishment with resulting physical harm, pain or mental anguish. Abuse also includes the deprivation by an individual, including a caretaker, of goods or services that are necessary to attain or maintain physical, mental, and psychosocial well-being. Instances of abuse of all residents, irrespective of any mental or physical condition, cause physical harm, pain, or mental anguish. It includes verbal abuse, sexual abuse, physical abuse, and mental abuse including abuse facilitated or enabled with technology. Willful, as used in this definition of abuse, means the individual must have acted deliberately, not that the individual must have intended to inflict injury or harm.

Accidents: an unforeseen and unplanned event or circumstance

Accommodation: resolving conflict by giving into wishes of another person

Accountable: Responsible to somebody or for something; capable of being explained

Accreditation: process of certifying that a facility meets certain quality and performance standards

Ache: to suffer a usually dull persistent pain

Acquired immunodeficiency syndrome (AIDS): severe disorder of the immune system caused by the human immunodeficiency virus (HIV)

Activities: the quality or state of being active

Activities Director/Coordinator: staff member who plans and directs activities for residents

Active-assistive ROM- the nurse assistant assists the resident in performing the exercise

Active Listening: deliberate effort to hear not only the words that another person is saying but, the complete message being communicated.

Activities of Daily Living (ADL): Shall mean one (1) or more of the following: Eating; Dressing; Bathing; Toileting; Transferring and Walking.

Active range of motion exercises: movement carried out by the resident

Acute: developing rapidly with pronounced symptoms and lasting a short time; rapid onset, short term duration

Acute Change of Condition: a sudden, deviation from a resident's baseline in physical, cognitive, behavioral, or functional domains

Acute pain: a sudden feeling of physical discomfort and distress and is usually the result of an accident, injury, or sudden illness (heart attack, appendicitis).

Addiction: a psychological and physical inability to stop consuming a chemical, drug, activity, or substance, even though it is causing psychological and physical harm

Adduction: toward the center (midline) of the body

Administrator: general manager of a facility

Admission: process of checking a person into a health care facility

Advance Directive: A document that designates the resident's wishes in the event that he/she is unable to speak for himself/herself

Adverse event. An adverse event is an untoward, undesirable, and usually unanticipated event that causes death or serious injury, or the risk thereof

Advocacy: support for or recommendation of a particular cause or policy. In health care patient advocacy can be a formal role assigned to someone specifically trained but all staff who care for the resident/patient are advocates for the person.

Advocate: a person who defends someone else

Afebrile: without fever

Affordable Care Act of 2010: The comprehensive health **care** reform law enacted in March **2010** (sometimes known as ACA, PPACA, or "**Obamacare**"). ... The law provides consumers with subsidies ("premium tax credits") that lower costs for households with incomes between 100% and 400% of the federal poverty level.

Agitation: vocal or motor behaviors such as shouting, fidgeting, pacing, screaming, or wandering

Agnosia: loss of the ability to recognize familiar objects

Aggressive: A type of behavior intending to cause physical or mental harm which can be hostile or violent. It may be reactionary and impulsive.

Aggressive Behavior: To consider one's self only with no consideration of another. *"I'm going to get my needs met even if it hurts you."*

Airborne precautions: measures taken to prevent the airborne transmission of pathogens

Airborne transmission: infection spread by microorganisms contained in particles or droplets suspended in the air

Altruism: belief in or practice of disinterested and selfless concern for the well-being of others.

Alveoli: any of the many tiny air sacs of the lungs which allow for rapid gaseous exchange

Alzheimer's Disease- a progress impairment of memory, reasoning, and judgement that is related to cellular changes within the brain and that leads to loss of independence in activities of daily living.

Anaphylactic Shock: an extreme, often life-threatening allergic reaction to an antigen to which the body has become hypersensitive.

Ambivalence: the state of having mixed feelings or contradictory ideas about something or someone.

Ambulate - To Move from One Place to Another

Ambulation: ability to walk

Ambulatory: able to walk

Analgesic: medicines that are used to relieve pain

Anterior: toward the front

Angina - Chest Pain

Antibiotic: drug that inhibits the growth of or kills certain microorganisms

Antibiotic resistant: describes microorganisms that have evolved in a way that makes them resistant to the action of antibiotics

Antibody: protein produced by the body to fight infection or illness

Anti-embolism stockings: elastic hosiery used to minimize the occurrence of edema and blood clots

Anus: outlet of the rectum

Anxiety: apprehensive uneasiness or nervousness usually over an impending or anticipated event. Intense, excessive, and persistent worry and fear about everyday situations. Often, anxiety disorders involve repeated episodes of sudden feelings of intense anxiety and fear or terror that reach a peak within minutes (panic attacks).

Aphasia: language difficulty due to brain damage, which can affect listening, speaking, reading and writing skills, loss of ability to use or understand language

Apical pulse: pulse taken at the apex of the heart

Apnea: cessation of breathing, during **apnea**, there is no movement of the muscles of inhalation, and the volume of the lungs initially remains unchanged.

Appetite: a natural desire to satisfy a bodily need, especially for food. Loss of appetite (anorexia) implies that hunger is absent—a person with anorexia has no desire to eat.

Apraxia: loss of ability to carry out planned movements at will (e.g. dressing, eating, bathing)

Arteries: blood vessels that carry blood away from the heart

Arteriosclerosis: loss of elasticity in the walls of the blood vessels

Arthritis: inflammation of a joint

Artificial airway: tubular devise placed into the respiratory tract to facilitate breathing or the removal of secretions

Asepsis: the absence of germs

Aseptic: free of microorganisms, preventing infection

Assertive Behavior: Placing yourself first but taking others into account. *"I will get my needs met and will not hurt you in the process."*

Aspiration/Aspirate: to draw fluid or object into the lung when breathing in, to suck in

Assault: threat or attempt to injure another in an unlawful manner.

Assessment: an appraisal of the whole person to establish a baseline and determine the resident's potential and his/her need for help

Asthma: a respiratory condition marked by spasms in the bronchi of the lungs, causing difficulty in breathing. It usually results from an allergic reaction or other forms of hypersensitivity.

Assisted Living Facility (ALF): Shall mean any premises, other than a residential care facility, intermediate care facility, or skilled nursing care facility, that is utilized by its owner, operator, or manager to provide twenty-four (24) hour care and services and protective oversight to three (3) or more residents who are provided with shelter, board, and who may need and are provided with the following:

(A) Assistance with any activities of daily living and any instrumental activities of daily living.

(B) Storage, distribution, or administration of medications; and

(C) Supervision of health care under the direction of a licensed physician, provided that such services are consistent with a social model of care.

(D) The term "assisted living facility" does not include a facility where all the residents are related within the fourth degree of consanguinity or affinity to the owner, operator, or manager of the facility.

Atherosclerosis: Accumulation of fat deposits inside of arteries, making them more narrow

Atom: the basic unit of a chemical element.

Atrophy: wasting away of muscle tissue leading to weakness, progressive decline

Aura: a sensation that often proceeds a seizure

Auscultation: using a stethoscope to hear sounds produced by internal organs (heart, lungs, bowels)

Automated External Defibrillator (AED): A portable device that can check a heart's rhythm and deliver a shock to the heart to restore a normal rhythm.

Autonomy: ability to act independently and make decisions for oneself

Avoidance: staying away from a person or issue instead of dealing with a conflict

Awareness: consciousness of one's environment

Axilla- armpit

B

Bacteria: single-celled organisms that can cause disease/illness

CNA: A Person-Centered Approach-Supplemental Manual

Basic Human Needs: activities required by all people to live their lives successfully and satisfactorily.

Baseline: initial measurement or observation used for later comparison

Battery: unlawful application of force to the person of another

Behavior: the way in which one acts or conducts oneself, especially toward others.

Behavioral: involving, relating to, or emphasizing behavior

Behavioral Symptoms: actions caused by a disease or condition. persistent or repetitive **behaviors** that are unusual, disruptive, inappropriate, or cause problems. Aggression, criminal **behavior**, defiance, drug use, hostility, inappropriate sexual **behavior**, inattention, secrecy, and self-harm are examples

Benign prostatic hyperplasia (BPH): enlargement of the prostate gland

Bereavement: period of mourning after the death of a loved one

Biohazardous waste: waste containing blood or other potentially infectious substances; including needles, blades, and other sharps

Bipolar Disorder: brain disorders that cause changes in a person's mood, energy and ability to function

Bladder: a muscular sac that stores the urine in the body

Bladder Diary: A bladder diary is a tool used to better understand bladder symptoms. It helps track a number of things: when and how much fluid is taken in, when and volume of urination, how often someone has that an urgency feeling, and when and how much urine may leak.

Blindness: inability to see

Blood Pressure: the amount of force exerted against the walls of an artery by the blood

Bloodshot: inflamed to redness

Bodily Discharge: something that is emitted, drainage from a body opening or wound

Body Language: nonverbal communication that includes posture, gestures, and facial expressions

Body Mass Index (BMI): measurement that estimates the percentage of fat tissue in the body

Body mechanics: using correct techniques in performing certain functions in a manner that does not add undue strain to the body

Body system: group of organs and structures that work together to perform vital functions

Body temperature: the amount of heat in the body that is a balance between the amount of heat produced and the amount lost by the body

Bony Prominence: Any point on the body where the bone is immediately below the

skin surface

Bowel movement: solid waste eliminated from the digestive tract

Bowel obstruction: a blockage in the intestine

Brace: device that supports and strengthens a body part

Brachial artery: the artery in the antecubital space in front of the elbow

Bradycardia: slow pulse rate, usually less than 60 beats per minute

Breach: an act of breaking or failing to observe a law, agreement, or code of conduct. A breach is, generally, an impermissible use or disclosure under the Privacy Rule that compromises the security or privacy of the protected health information. A server where the information is stored is breached.

Bronchi: two large branches of the trachea through which air moves in and out of the lungs

Bronchioles: branches of each bronchus

Bronchitis: Bronchitis is an inflammation of the bronchial tubes, the airways that carry air to your lungs. It causes a cough that often brings up mucus. It can also cause shortness of breath, wheezing, a low fever, and chest tightness. There are two main types of bronchitis: acute and chronic.

C

Call System (call bell, call light): in the patient unit, this consists of a signal cord or button. This signal activates a bell, light, or intercom system used to request assistance. The cord or button must be always placed within the patient's reach.

Calorie: A unit of food energy.

Cannula: a plastic or metal tube

Cancer: group of diseases characterized by the uncontrolled growth of abnormal cells

Carbohydrates: any of a large group of organic compounds occurring in foods and living tissues and including sugars, starch, and cellulose. They contain hydrogen and oxygen in the same ratio as water (2:1) and typically can be broken down to release energy in the body.

Cardiac Arrest: complete cessation of heart activity (no heartbeat/pulse)

Cardiopulmonary resuscitation (CPR): emergency procedure to restore cardiopulmonary function

Care Area Assessment (CAA): . The CAA process provides a framework for guiding the review of triggered areas, and clarification of a resident's functional status and related causes of impairments. It also provides a basis for additional assessment of potential issues, including related risk factors. The assessment of the causes and contributing factors gives the interdisciplinary team (IDT) additional information to help them develop a comprehensive plan of care.

Care Plan: an individual plan of care for each resident. The facility must develop a comprehensive care plan for each resident that includes measurable objectives and timetables to meet a resident's medical, nursing, and mental and psychosocial needs that are identified in the comprehensive assessment. The care plan must describe the following:

> (i) The services that are to be furnished to attain or maintain the resident's highest practicable physical, mental, and psychosocial well-being as required and
>
> (ii) Any services that would otherwise be required but are not provided due to the resident's exercise of rights under including the right to refuse treatment under

Caring: Compassionate or showing concern for others, belonging or relating to a profession that involves looking after people's physical, medical, or general welfare, e.g. nursing or social work, provision of medical or other types of care, either professionally or in general

Cataract: clouding of the lens of the eye

Catastrophic reaction: overreaction to circumstances

Catheter: a sterile tube inserted into the bladder to drain urine

Cells: Cells are the basic units of all living things. The human body is made of trillions of cells. There are many different types of cells and each has a special function.

Centers for Medicare and Medicaid Services: (CMS): The Centers for Medicare & Medicaid Services, CMS, is part of the Department of Health and Human Services (HHS) and is responsible for enforcing regulations in America's nursing homes.

Cerebral vascular accident (CVA): condition that occurs when blood flow to the brain is interrupted; also called a stroke

Certified Medication Technician: Trained and certified nurse assistants who are, once certified, able to administer nonparental medications and assist licensed practical nurses or registered professional nurses in medication therapy. (Not recognized in every state)

Chain of infection: process by which infection is spread

Change of Condition: see acute change of condition or significant change of condition

Character: The set of qualities that make somebody or something distinctive, especially somebody's qualities of mind and feeling, qualities that make somebody or something interesting or attractive. Knowing the good, loving the good and doing the good. "*The ability to gain control of personal desires, develop a deep regard for others, put aside personal interests and needs to serve others*".

Charge nurse: nursing professional with day-to-day responsibility for supervising resident care

"**Chemical restraint**" is defined as any drug that is used for discipline or staff convenience and not required to treat medical symptoms.

Chemotherapy: type of drug therapy used as a treatment for disease, especially cancer

Cheyne-Stokes: a pattern of breathing in which respirations gradually increase in rate and depth and then become shallow and slow, breathing may stop for 10 to 20 seconds

Cheerfulness: Having a pleasant and happy nature; smiling frequently and communicating effectively with co-workers. A happy and optimistic mood, or happy and optimistic by nature causing people to feel cheerful showing willingness or good humor in complying.

Chills: a sensation of cold accompanied by shivering (as due to illness)

Cholesterol: fatty substance produced by the body and ingested in food

Chronic: continuing over a long period of time or recurring frequently; chronic conditions begin insidiously, and symptoms are not as noticeable as in acute conditions, long, drawn out, long term.

Chronic Kidney Disease: a type of kidney disease in which there is gradual loss of kidney function over a period of months to years. Initially there are generally no symptoms; later, symptoms may include leg swelling, feeling tired, vomiting, loss of appetite, and confusion. Complications include an increased risk of heart disease, high blood pressure, bone disease, and anemia.

Chronic obstructive pulmonary disease (COPD): chronic inflammatory disease of the bronchial passages and lungs; there most common types are bronchitis, emphysema and asthma

Chronic pain is pain that is ongoing and usually lasts longer than six months.

Circulatory system: body system that includes the heart, blood vessels, and lymphatic tissues and vessels

Circumcision- a surgical removal of the end of the foreskin of the penis

Citation: includes: (1) the alpha prefix and data tag number, (2) the Code of Federal Regulations (CFR), or Life Safety Page 4 Code (LSC) **reference**, (3) the language from that **reference** which pinpoints the aspect(s) of the requirement with which the entity (Facility) failed to do or assure.

Clarity: clearness of communication

Cleaning: removing soil from a surface or object

Clostridium difficile: spore-forming bacterium which can cause infection known as ***Clostridium difficile* infection (CDI).** Symptoms include watery diarrhea, fever, nausea, and abdominal pain. It makes up about 20% of cases of antibiotic-associated diarrhea

Code of Ethics: A code of ethics is a guide of principles designed to help professionals conduct business honestly and with integrity. A code of ethics also referred to as an "ethical code," may encompass areas such as business ethics, a code of professional practice and an employee code of conduct.

Code of Federal Regulation (CFR): set of rules published in the Federal Register by departments and agencies of the U.S, government

Coccyx: the bone at the base of the spine (tailbone)

Coercion: the practice of persuading someone to do something by using force or threats.

Cognitive: dealing with the thoughts and emotions

Cognitive ability: The ability of the brain to process, retrieve, and store information. Impairment of these brain functions is common in patients with dementia, drug intoxication, or head injury.

Cognitive impairment: measurable decline in memory and thinking skills

Collaboration: working together to accomplish a task or resolve a conflict

Colostomy: an artificial opening made in the abdominal wall to allow the passage of feces through a stoma (opening)

Comatose: describes a person who is in a coma (unconscious)

Combativeness: physically aggressive behavior, hitting, kicking, scratching, biting

Common area: Common areas are areas in the facility where residents may gather together with other residents, visitors, and staff or engage in individual pursuits, apart from their residential rooms. This includes but is not limited to living rooms, dining rooms, activity rooms, outdoor areas, and meeting rooms where residents are located on a regular basis.

Communication: The exchange of information between people, e.g. by means of speaking, writing, or using a common system of signs or behavior, the communicating of information

Communication Skills: Learned skills which help a person communicate more effectively. Such as listening, asking questions for clarity, etc.

Commitment: the state or quality of being dedicated to a cause, activity, etc.

Compassionate: Showing feelings of sympathy for the suffering of others, often with a desire to help

Competency: the ability to properly perform a specific task

Competition: the activity or condition of competing.

Complaint Survey: A survey to investigate formal complaints received by the survey agency.

Compliance: The action or fact of complying with a wish, command, law or regulation.

Compromise: resolving conflict by both parties agreeing to something less or different that they originally wanted to achieve a peaceful resolution

Conscience: an inner feeling or voice viewed as acting as a guide to the rightness or wrongness of one's behavior. *"He had a **guilty conscience** about his desires."*

Condom catheter: an external catheter applied to males (Texas catheter)

Conduct: one's actions in general; behavior

Confidence: the feeling or belief that one can rely on someone or something; firm trust

Confidential: personal, not known to others

Confidentiality: Carried out or revealed in the expectation that anything done or revealed will be kept private, entrusted with somebody's personal or private matters, not available to the public, e.g., because it is protected medical information

Conflict: a serious disagreement or argument. A conflict is a clash of interest.

Conflict Resolution is the process of finding a peaceful solution to a disagreement or argument or reduction in the severity of a disagreement or argument

Confused: state of being mixed up

Constant: marked by firm steadfast resolution or faithfulness

Continence: the ability to retain a bodily discharge voluntarily

Confusion: a mental state characterized by disorientation regarding time, place or person

Congestive heart failure (CHF): the inability of the heart to pump an adequate quantity of blood

Consent: permission granted voluntarily by a person in his/her (sound/clear) mind

Consensual Relationship shall **mean** and refer to any **relationship**, either past or present, which is romantic, intimate, or sexual in nature and to which both parties' consent or consented.

Consenting resident means a resident whose participation in an intimate relationship or sexual activity is volitional.

Consistency: degree of firmness, density, viscosity, or resistance to movement or separation of constituent particles

Constipation: the passage of unusually dry, hard stool

Constrict: get smaller

Contact precautions: measure taken to prevent the spread of infection caused by microorganisms transmitted by direct or indirect contact

Context: the entire situation, background, or environment that provides meaning to a person's words

Contaminated: exposed to germs

Continuity of Care: A continuous relationship between a patient and an identified health-care professional who is the sole source of care and information for the patient. However, as a patient's healthcare needs over time can rarely be met by a single professional, multi-professional pathways of continuity exist to achieve both quality of care and patient satisfaction.

Continuing care retirement community: facility that provides several tiers of care; independent living, assisted living, and skilled nursing care

Contracture: shortening of muscles and tendons, which causes deformity of joint and a decrease in joint motion and muscle wasting

Convenience: result of any action that has the effect of altering a resident's behavior such that the resident requires a lesser amount of effort or care and is not in the resident's best interest.

Coronary artery disease (CAD): condition in which the major blood vessels that supply the heart become damaged or diseased, often due to plaque build-up and/or inflammation

Cuing: prompting a resident to begin a task or activity by telling or showing

Culture: the collection customs, attitudes, and beliefs of a particular group of people; may relate to ethnic or religious background and/or social groups

Contusion: an injury that does not break the skin, caused by a blow to the body and characterized by swelling, discoloration, and pain

Cultural Competency: refers to the ability for healthcare professionals to demonstrate cultural competence toward patients with diverse values, beliefs, and feelings. This process includes consideration of the individual social, cultural, and psychological needs of patients. The goal of cultural competence in health care is to reduce health disparities and to provide optimal care to patients regardless of their race, gender, ethnic background, native languages spoken, and religious or cultural beliefs.

Cultural safety: the effective nursing practice of a person or family from another culture that is determined by that person or family. Its origins are in nursing education and a culture can range anywhere from age or generation, gender, sexual orientation, occupation, religious beliefs, or even disabilities.

Courage: The ability to face danger, difficulty, uncertainty, or pain without being overcome by fear or being deflected from a chosen course of action. "*Acquire the ability to overcome or endure difficulties, including pain, inconvenience, disappointment, setbacks, worry and boredom. Get in the habit of overcoming anxiety or fear through purposeful, honorable action.*"

Customer service: the actions involved in serving a customer's needs

Customs: traditional practices of a particular group of people

Cyanotic/Cycosis: a bluish-gray color of the skin, lips, or nail beds due to lack of oxygen

Cystic Fibrosis: is a genetic disorder that affects mostly the lungs, but also the pancreas, liver, kidneys, and intestine. Long-term issues include difficulty breathing and coughing up mucus because of frequent lung infections. Other signs and symptoms may include sinus infections, poor growth, fatty stool, clubbing of the fingers and toes, and infertility in most males

D

Dangle: to sit on the side of the bed with the legs over the edge of the mattress

Deafness: inability to hear

Death: a natural part of life where all vital functions of the body cease

Decubitus Ulcer: an inflammation, sore, or lesion that develops over areas where the skin and tissue underneath are injured due to a lack of blood flow

Deep Tissue Injury: A pressure-related **injury** to subcutaneous **tissues** under intact skin

Defecation: passing feces from the body; passing of stool

Deficiency: in regard to the survey process a deficiency is a written notice of inadequate care or sub-standard practice usually based around a facilities failure to do or provide care or items required by regulation

Defensiveness: being overly sensitive to perceived criticism from others

Dehydration: loss of body's normal water content, which can affect both physical and mental functions

Delegate: entrust (a task or responsibility) to another person, typically one who is less senior than oneself but not always.

Delusion: false thought that a person believes to be real

Delirium: memory and thinking impairment that comes on suddenly and is caused by illness or toxic reactions in the body, usually reversible

Demeanor is defined as the way a person acts toward other people including behavior, conduct and appearance.

Dementia: severe impairment of cognitive functions such as thinking, memory, and personally; comes on slowly and worsens over time; usually irreversible, depending on the cause of the dementia

Denial: avoiding an issue or problem instead of dealing with it directly

Dentures: artificial, or false teeth

Dependent: unable to care for one's self

Depression: a mood disorder that causes a persistent feeling of sadness and loss of interest.

Dermatitis: inflammation of the skin

Dermis: inner layer of the skin beneath the epidermis

Developmental disability: chronic condition caused by physical and/or mental impairment that affects language, learning, mobility, and the activities of daily living independently

Diabetes: a chronic disease characterized by insufficient insulin production or utilization

Diagnosis: determining what kind of disease or medical condition a person has, the information should be in the patient's chart, the doctor determines diagnosis based on tests, observations, etc.

Dialysis: process of filtering and removing waste products from the blood used when the kidneys are not functioning properly

Diaphoresis: excessive sweating

Diarrhea: frequent passage of liquid stool

Diastolic pressure: the pressure in the arteries when the heart is at rest (the bottom number of the blood pressure reading)

Digestion: process by which food is broken down, mechanically and chemically and changed to a form that can be absorbed by the body

Digestive System: body system involved in processing food, providing nutrients to the body, and expelling waste

Dignity: The condition of being worthy of respect, esteem, or honor. *Respecting the dignity of residents and others.*

Dilate: to get larger

Direct Transmission: spread of infection from one person to another or when infected blood or body fluids come in direct contact with broken skin or mucous membranes

Director of Nursing: senior nursing professional who directs the approach for care and determines staffing requirements

Discharge: the resident goes to another facility such as a hospital or other long-term care facility, home or to another person's home, or if the resident dies.

Discriminate: To recognize a distinction or to differentiate.

Disinfection: process that kills or inhibits the growth of virtually all microorganisms on objects and surfaces

Discipline: is defined as any action taken by the facility for the purpose of punishing or penalizing residents.

Disciplinary Action: Concerning or enforcing discipline and can include censure, fine, suspension, or expulsion. **Disciplinary procedures** are used to punish individuals for violating the rules, policies, procedures, or professional codes of conduct.

Disorientation: the state of mental confusion or loss of bearings in relation to the sense of person, place, or time

Distention: the state of being inflated or enlarged

Diversionary: to draw attention to something else or to amuse

Diversity: the state of variety and the practice or quality of including or involving people from a range of different social and ethnic backgrounds and of different genders, sexual orientations, etc..

Documentation: written and/or digital reports maintained by the facility relating to a residents' care and condition

Dull: lacking sharpness of edge or point

Durable power of attorney for healthcare: a written authorization to represent or act on another's behalf in private affairs, business, or some other legal matter. For our purposes we are talking about medical decisions not legal, financial or other forms of legal power of attorney. The person authorizing the other to act is the principal, grantor, or donor (of the power). The one authorized to act is the agent, attorney, or in some common law jurisdictions, the attorney-in-fact.

Droplet spread measures taken to prevent the spread of infection caused by microorganisms transmitted by

Dysarthria: weakness or paralysis of muscles off lips, tongue, and throat; may be due to brain damage from stroke or accident.

Dysphagia: difficulty swallowing

Dyspnea: difficulty in breathing

E

Eating Disorder: a mental disorder defined by abnormal eating habits that negatively affect a person's physical or mental health.

Electronic medical record: digital version of the patient chart and medical record

Edema: swelling due to an accumulation of watery fluid in the tissue

Electronic Healthcare Record: the systematized collection of patient and population electronically stored health information in a digital format. These records can be shared across different health care settings.

Element: each of more than one hundred substances that cannot be chemically interconverted or broken down into simpler substances and are primary constituents of matter. Each element is distinguished by its atomic number, i.e., the number of protons in the nuclei of its atoms.

Elder Justice Act of 2010: The EJA applies to seniors aged 60 or older and is the first piece of comprehensive national legislation to address elder abuse. One of its objectives is to coordinate responses to elder abuse across federal and state agencies and to support efforts to detect and prevent elder abuse. The EJA seeks to promote elder justice, which it defines as efforts to "prevent, detect, treat, intervene in, and prosecute elder abuse, neglect and exploitation [and] protect elders with diminished capacity while maximizing their autonomy."

Elimination: to rid the body of wastes, such as urine or stool

Elopement: also known as wandering, in the nursing home setting refers to the patient leaving a facility without notice or staff awareness

Emesis: vomiting

Emotion: one's feelings

Emotional Awareness: Emotional awareness is the ability to recognize and make sense of not just your own emotions, but also those of others.

Empathy: ability to understand and share the feelings or perspective of another person

Emphysema: respiratory condition in which the elasticity of the alveoli is lost, resulting in difficulty breathing

Endocrine System: body system made up of glands that secrete hormones

Endorphins: natural morphine-like substances produced by the nervous system that reduce the sensation of pain

Enema: a procedure in which liquid or gas is injected into the rectum, typically to expel its contents, but also to introduce drugs or permit X-ray imaging or other procedures

Enteral nutrition: providing liquid nourishment using a nasogastric tube or a tube surgically inserted through the abdominal wall into the stomach

Epidermis: surface (outer) layer of the skin

Equality: the state of being equal, especially in status, rights, and opportunities.

Esophagus: a tube connecting the throat to the stomach through which food passes

Ethical: relating to a set of moral principles and values

Ethical decision making is the process in which you aim to make your decisions in line with a code of ethics.

Ethics: the discipline that addresses what is good and bad and what is moral duty and obligation

Ethical Behavior: Acting in ways consistent with what society and individuals typically think are good values.

Evaluate: to decide if a course of action was the correct one to take

Eversion: a turning outward

Expectorate: coughing up matter from respiratory tract and spitting it out

Exploitation: illegal or improper use of a person's property or resources to the degree that substantial risk of harm exists

Exposure: being in the vicinity of or in contact with an infectious microorganism

Extended Survey: The **Extended Survey** is conducted when there is a finding of substandard quality of care during a standard **survey**. The **extended survey** includes: The review of a larger sample of resident assessments. The review of staffing & in-service training.

Extension: to straighten; to extend
External customer: residents, family, and customers who are outside of the long-term care facility

External Evacuation: moving residents out of the facility to another site for safety

External rotation: to move the extremity in a circular motion away from the center of the body

Extremities: the arms, legs, hands, and feet

Exploitation. Exploitation means taking advantage of a resident for personal gain using manipulation, intimidation, threats, or coercion.

F

Face sheet: one-page summary of important identifying information regarding a patient or resident

False imprisonment: unjustified detention of a person

Fatigued: drained of strength and energy

Fats: a natural oily or greasy substance occurring in animal bodies, especially when deposited as a layer under the skin or around certain organs.

Febrile: feverish

Fecal Impaction: a solid, immobile bulk of feces that can develop in the rectum as a result of chronic constipation

Feces: waste products in the bowel; same as stool or BM

Fever: elevation of body temperature above the normal

Five Star Rating System: CMS created the Five-Star Quality Rating System to help consumers, their families, and caregivers compare nursing homes more easily and to help identify areas about which they may want to ask questions. The Nursing Home Compare Web site features a quality rating system that gives each nursing home a rating of between 1 and 5 stars. Nursing homes with 5 stars are considered to have much above average quality and nursing homes with 1 star are considered to have quality much below average.

- physical and clinical needs.

Fixed: not subject to change or fluctuation. When we talk about fixed pupils they do not follow movement and do not respond to light.

Flatus: gas in the bowel

Flexion: to bend

Flow sheet: document used to record health and activity information about a resident over a period

Flushed: reddened color of the skin

Foot board: a piece of wood or plastic at the end of the bed for positioning the resident's feet

Foot cradle: a metal or plastic frame over the foot of the bed that lifts the weight of the sheets off of the resident's feet

Foreskin: loose skin at and covering the end of the penis

Fowler's Position: lying on the back with the head of the bed elevated 45 to 60 degrees

Fracture: a broken bone

Freedom of movement: any change in place or position for the body or any part of the body that the person is physically able to control.

F-TAG: Federal Regulatory Groups for Long-Term Care Facilities. The tag number corresponds with the topic of the regulation; F684 regards Quality of Care at 483.25 (location of federal regulation.

Functional incontinence: leakage in the presence of an intact lower urinary tract system and is due to functional limitations such as decreased mobility, cognitive impairment,

Fungus: type of microorganism that can cause infection; (yeast and mold)

G

Gait: a manner of walking or moving on foot, a sequence of foot movements (such as a walk, trot, pace, or canter) by which a horse or a dog moves forward, a manner or rate of movement or progress

Gait Belt: canvas belt placed around the resident's waist to assist with ambulation and transfers
Gangrene: death of tissue usually due to deficient or absent blood supply

Genes: a unit of heredity which is transferred from a parent to offspring and is held to determine some characteristic of the offspring.

Genetic: relating to genes or heredity

Gerontology: science field focused on the study of aging

Germ: microorganism

Gingivitis: inflammation of the gums.

Glaucoma: increase of pressure within the eye, resulting in blindness if left untreated

Graduate: a container marked with lines for measuring liquids

Goals: Something that somebody wants to achieve; a desired result or outcome

Grievance: formal complaint of a wrong, injury or injustice

Grimace: a facial expression usually of disgust, disapproval, or pain

Guarding: the act or duty of protecting or defending, a defensive position

H

Halitosis: bad breath

Hallucination: sensory perceptions that seem real to the person experiencing them but are not perceived by others

HIPPA: Health Insurance Portability and Accountability Act). A 1996 Federal law that restricts access to individuals' private medical information. It protects personal healthcare information of patients and prohibits care providers from disclosing that information without the express written permission of the patient.

Healthcare related infection (HAI): infection contracted while an inpatient, outpatient or in a residential health care facility

Heart attack/myocardial infarction (MI): a blockage or clot occurring in an artery in the heart, resulting in chest pain due to tissue damage

Heimlich Maneuver: emergency procedure to dislodge food or object obstructing the airway

Hemiplegia: loss of sensation or movement in one side of the body

Hemodialysis: type of dialysis in which the blood is removed from the body and filtered through a machine that removes waste products and excess fluid and returns the blood to the body

Hemorrhage: excessive, uncontrolled bleeding
Hemorrhoids: varicose veins in the rectum that can be painful, itch and bleed
Hepatitis: viral infection of the liver

History: The events and experiences of an individual's past

History and Physical(H&P): patient/resident history combined with a physical examination

Hives: an allergic disorder marked by raised edematous patches of skin or mucous membrane and usually intense itching and caused by contact with a specific precipitating factor (such as a food, drug, or inhalant) either externally or internally

Honesty: Always truthful and genuine; demonstrating good work ethics. The quality, condition, or characteristic of being fair, truthful, and morally upright, truthfulness, candor, or sincerity

Hormones: a regulatory substance produced in an organism and transported in tissue fluids such as blood or sap to stimulate specific cells or tissues into action.

Hospice: a type of care that provides comfort for terminally ill persons

Hospice care: care provided to meet the physical, emotional, and spiritual needs of patients with terminal illness and their families

Human immunodeficiency virus (HIV): virus that attacks the body's immune system

Hydration: supplying water to the body to maintain fluid balance

Hygiene: personal cleanliness

Hyperactivity: the state or condition of being overly active

Hyperextension: extensive extension

Hyperglycemia: high blood sugar

Hypoactivity: less than normally active

Hypodermis: layer of fatty tissue beneath the epidermis

Hypoglycemia: low blood sugar

Hypertension: high blood pressure, condition in which systolic BP is above 150 mm HG and Diastolic is above 90 mm Hg

Hypotension: low blood pressure, condition in which systolic BP is below 100 mm HG and Diastolic is below 60 mm Hg

Hypothermia: when the temperature of the body is below the individual's normal range

Hypoxia: state in which there is not enough oxygen reaching body tissues

I

Incentive Spirometer: a device that measures how deeply you can inhale (breathe in). It helps you take slow, deep breaths to expand and fill your lungs with air. This helps prevent lung problems, such as pneumonia. The **incentive spirometer** is made up of a breathing tube, an air chamber, and an indicator

Immunization: administration of a vaccine to prevent a specific infectious disease

Impairment: An objective handicap, partial disability, loss of function, anatomic or functional defect, which may be temporary or permanent persisting after appropriate therapy, without reasonable prospect of improvement, ranging from mild to severe

Intake and Output (I & O): to measure and record all liquids ingested and expelled by a patient

Involuntary movement: Movement that is not subject to control.

Immobility: unable to move

Impaction: hard stool that cannot pass from the rectum normally

Incident Report: a form that is filled out to record details of an unusual event that occurs at the facility, such as an accident with or without injury. The purpose of the incident report is to document the exact details of the occurrence while they are fresh in the minds of those who witnessed the event. It may also be used for tracking and reporting to Quality Assurance or Safety Committees.

Incontinent: inability to control the passage of urine

Independent: self-reliant, able to care for oneself

Individualized Care: Individualized care is considered an important indicator of quality nursing care. Knowing the patient has been described as the process by which nurses come to understand their patient's experiences, behaviors, feelings and perceptions to individualize their care.

Indwelling urinary catheter: a sterile tube inserted through the urethra into the bladder to drain urine; held in place by a small, inflated balloon.

Infection: invasion of the body by a disease producing (pathogen) microorganism

Infectious agent is the pathogen (germ) that causes diseases.

Inflammation: a local response to cellular injury that is marked by capillary dilatation, leukocytic infiltration, redness, heat, and pain and that serves as a mechanism initiating the elimination of noxious agents and of damaged tissue

Influenza: viral respiratory infection; also called the flu

In-service education: educational programs provided for employees while on the job CNA's are required to have at least 12 hours per year after initial certification.

Inhale: to breathe in

Insomnia: habitual sleeplessness; inability to sleep

Insubordination: Refusing to obey orders or submit to authority

Itching: an uneasy irritating sensation in the upper surface of the skin usually held to result from mild stimulation of pain receptors

Intake and Output (I &O): Intake is the act of consuming or taking in of food, fluids, or substances into the body. Output is the process of waste exiting the body.

Integumentary System: body system made up of the skin, nail and hair

Interim Survey: a revisit survey following up on previous deficiencies found in the annual survey.

Intermediate Care Facility (ICF): A facility that **Interdisciplinary team:** staff members from various departments who work together to plan and implement care provides 24-hour room, board, personal care and basic health and nursing care services to three or more residents. The care is provided under the daily supervision of a licensed nurse and under the direction of a licensed doctor.

Internal evacuation: moving residents to another location within the facility for safety also known as lateral evacuation

Internal Rotation: to move the extremity in a circular motion toward the center of the body

Interdisciplinary Team: a group of people or units organized to do a task together. In healthcare an interdisciplinary team is a group of health care professionals from diverse fields who work in a coordinated fashion toward common goals for the patient/resident

Intervention: The action or process of intervening to affect an outcome toward the positive.

Intimacy: An expression of the natural desire of human persons for connection; a state of reciprocated physical closeness to, and emotional honesty with, another. Physical closeness to another includes physical touch as demonstrated by nongenital, nonsexual touching, hugging, and caressing. Intimacy is not a synonym for sex; however, sexual activity frequently occurs within an intimate relationship.

Invasion of Privacy: a civil wrong that unlawfully makes public knowledge of any private or personal information without the consent of the wronged person.

Inversion: a turning inward (feet only)

Involuntary seclusion: Defined as separation of a resident from other residents or from her/his room or confinement to her/his room (with or without roommates) against the resident's will, or the will of the resident's legal representative. Emergency or short term monitored separation from other Residents will not be considered involuntary seclusion and may be permitted if used for a limited period as a therapeutic intervention to reduce agitation until professional staff can develop a plan of care to meet the resident's needs.

Isolation precautions: measures taken to prevent the spread of infection from an infected resident to other people

J

Jaundice: yellow discoloration of skin due to bile

Judgment: The ability to form sound opinions and make sensible decisions or reliable guesses

Justice: Being fair and having a commitment to others. Fairness or reasonableness, especially in the way people are treated or decisions are made

K

Ketones: substances made when the body breaks down fat for energy

Kidneys: filtering system of the body

Kiosk: centrally located electronic device used to input patient/resident data

L

Labia: the skin folds that are on both sides of the urethra and vagina

Laceration: wound produced by cutting or tearing

Larynx: the voice box

Latent: in a resting or dormant state

Lateral: to the side, side of the body

Legal: relating to the law

Legal Representative: a person appointed by a court to administer the estate of another person or to make decisions for another person, unable to do so themselves, such as medical decisions.

Leukemia: a malignant progressive disease in which the bone marrow and other blood-forming organs produce increased numbers of immature or abnormal leukocytes. These suppress the production of normal blood cells, leading to anemia and other symptoms.

Level of care: classification based on the intensity of medical and nursing services provided in a health care setting

Libel: a false and malicious publication in writing about an individual or group to a third party

Licensed health professional: A licensed health professional is a physician; physician assistant; nurse practitioner; physical, speech, or occupational therapist; physical or occupational therapy assistant; registered professional nurse; licensed practical nurse; or licensed or certified social worker; or registered respiratory therapist or certified respiratory therapy technician.

Licensed practical nurse (LPN) or licensed vocational nurse (LVN) : An individual who has completed a state-approved practical or vocational nursing program, passed the NCLEX-PN Examination, and is licensed by a state board of nursing to provide patient care. Normally works under the supervision of a registered nurse, advanced practice registered nurse or physician.

Licensed Social Worker (LSW): licensed professional who usually has a master's degree in social work who counsels residents and families

Limp: not stiff or rigid, lacking in strength, vigor, or firmness, to walk favoring one leg

Listen: To pay attention to something and take it into account, to concentrate on hearing somebody or something, an act of trying to hear something. *Yes, you heard me, but did you listen?*

Living Will: legal document that specifies a person's wishes in regard to withdrawing or withholding life-sustaining procedures and directs the medical treatments a person will accept or reject

Localized: confined to a local area of the body (one area)

Logrolling - Rolling Patients to the Side

Long-term care: a range of medical and nonmedical services provided for people who have a chronic illness, disability, or cognitive impairment that affects their ability to perform everyday tasks

Long-Term Care Ombudsman seeks to improve the quality of life for residents of long-term care facilities. These facilities include nursing homes, personal care homes and assisted living facilities. In addition, Ombudsmen serve residents who live in community living arrangements (CLAs) and intermediate care facilities for persons with mental retardation (ICF/MRs).

M

Macronutrient: a type of food (e.g. fat, protein, carbohydrate) required in large amounts in the diet.

Malignant: cancerous tumor or cells that grow uncontrollably and spread to other parts of the body

Malpractice: improper or negligent treatment of a resident or patient resulting in damage or injury.

Managed Care: type of health insurance coverage that monitors quality of care and is designed to contain costs

Manipulation: The usage of underhanded influence over a person, event, or situation to gain a desired outcome.

"**Manual method**" to hold or limit a resident's voluntary movement by using body contact as a method of physical restraint.

Material Safety Data Sheets (MDSD): A safety data sheet (SDS), material safety data sheet (MSDS), or product safety data sheet (PSDS) are documents that list information relating to occupational safety and health for the use of various substances and products. SDSs are a widely used system for cataloging information on chemicals, chemical compounds, and chemical mixtures. SDS information may include instructions for the safe use and potential hazards associated with a particular material or product, along with spill-handling procedures. The older MSDS formats could vary from source to source within a country depending on national requirements; however, the newer SDS format is internationally standardized.

MDS coordinator: staff member who assesses residents' functional capabilities and determines appropriate level of care

Meatus: opening in the urethra on the body surface through which urine is discharged

Medicaid: joint federal-state health insurance program for low-income individuals

Medical director: senior staff physician who directs medical care in a facility

Medical Record: the systematic documentation of a single patient's medical history and care across time within one health care provider's jurisdiction. Also known, interchangeably as health record, medical chart, clinical record, or electronic health record (EHR).

Medical symptom" an indication or characteristic of a physical or psychological condition.

Medicare: federal health insurance program for individuals age 65 and older and certain people with disabilities

Membranes: a thin sheet of tissue or layer of cells acting as a boundary, lining, or partition in an organism.

Mental abuse: Includes, but is not limited to, humiliation, harassment, threats of punishment or deprivation.

Mentally competent: capable of rational decision making and being responsible for one's actions

Mental and psychosocial adjustment difficulty: the development of emotional and/or behavioral symptoms in response to an identifiable stressor(s) that has not been the resident's typical response to stressors in the past or an inability to adjust to stressors as evidenced by chronic emotional and/or behavioral symptoms.

Mental Illness: behavioral or mental pattern that causes significant distress or impairment of personal functioning

Metabolism: the chemical processes that occur within a living organism in order to maintain life.

Metastasis: the spread of cancer cells to other parts of the body.

Micro: small

Micronutrients: a chemical element or substance required in trace amounts for the normal growth and development of living organisms (vitamins and minerals)

Microorganism: a very small living thing (a germ) that can only be seen with a microscope

Micturition – Urinating

Milliliter (ml)- same as cubic centimeter (cc)

Minerals: a chemical element required as an essential nutrient by organisms to perform functions necessary for life. The five major minerals in the human body are calcium, phosphorus, potassium, sodium, and magnesium.

Minimum Data System (MDS): The Minimum Data Set (**MDS**) is part of a federally mandated process for clinical **assessment** of all residents in Medicare or Medicaid certified nursing homes. This process entails a comprehensive, standardized **assessment** of each resident's functional capabilities and health needs.

Misappropriation of resident property: the deliberate misplacement, exploitation, or wrongful, temporary, or permanent use of a resident's belongings or money without the resident's consent

Mistreatment: inappropriate treatment or exploitation of a resident.

Mixed incontinence: the combination of urge and stress incontinence

mm Hg: millimeters of mercury, the unit of measurement used when taking blood pressure

Mobility: ability to move freely

Mode of transmission: how microorganisms is transferred from one carrier to another

Molecule: a group of atoms bonded together, representing the smallest fundamental unit of a chemical compound that can take part in a chemical reaction

Morals: one's own personal values which are concerned with the principles of right and wrong behavior and the goodness or badness of human character.

Mucous membranes: tissues that secrete mucous in nose, mouth

Mucus: sticky substance secreted by mucus membranes mainly in the lungs, nose, and parts of the rectal and genital areas

Multiple sclerosis: progressive disease that affects nerve fibers

Musculoskeletal system: body system made up of bones, muscles, tendons, ligaments, and joints

N

Neglect: failure of the facility, its employees or service providers to provide goods and services to a resident that are necessary to avoid physical harm, pain, mental anguish, or emotional distress.

Negligence: failure to perform in a reasonably prudent manner or by acceptable health care practices/standards

Nervous System: body system made up of brain, spinal cord and nerves

Nocturia: the need to urinate at night

Nonassertive Behavior: Put others before one's self. *"Your needs are important; my needs don't count."*

Non-Compliance: The facility was not in compliance with the specific regulatory requirement(s) (as referenced by the specific F-tag or K-tag) at the time the situation occurred; The facility was not following state or federal regulations.

Nonconsensual: not agreed to by one or more of the people involved. In sexual abuse even if a resident seems to enjoy the relationship if they do have the cognitive ability to consent it is nonconsensual.

Nonintact skin: skin that is broken, chapped, or cracked

Nonpathogenic: describes microorganisms that do not cause infection

Nonpharmalogical: Managing pain, behaviors, or other symptoms without medication.

Nonverbal communication: sending and receiving messages without using words

Nosocomial Infection: an infection acquired after admission to the facility (*If an infection starts at home it is not a nosocomial infection. If it starts in the healthcare environment (facility/hospital, etc. It is a nosocomial infection.)*

Nurse aide: A nurse aide is any individual providing nursing or nursing-related services to residents in a facility. This term may also include an individual who provides these services through an agency or under a contract with the facility, but is not a licensed health professional, a registered dietitian, or someone who volunteers to provide such services without pay. Nurse aides do not include those individuals who furnish services to residents only as paid feeding assistants as defined in §488.30

Nursing process: a problem-solving technique that consists of eight steps: (1) data collection, (2) assessment, (3) problem, (4) need, (5) goal, (6) approach, (7) implementation and (8) evaluation or outcome

Nursing Staff: The largest department in a long-term care facility and in most health care settings. The nursing staff are responsible for helping residents with activities of daily living, medical treatments, medications and the promotion and maintenance of health. The nursing department includes (RN's, LPNs, CNA's)

Nutrient: food that supplies the body with its necessary elements

Nutrition: the process of taking in food and energy from it

O

Obese: a status with body weight that is grossly above the acceptable or desirable weight, usually due to accumulation of excess fats in the body.

Objective: way to reach goal

Objective Information: factual information gathered through observation

Observations: the action or process of observing something or someone carefully or in order to gain information.

Observation Skills: Always on the lookout for anything unusual or significant. "*The resident seems confused today and warm to touch. The CNA notes these facts, secures the residents vital signs and reports to the charge nurse that there is something unusual with the resident.*"

Obstruction: a blockage

Occupational Safety and Health Administration (OSHA): federal agency responsible for protecting worker health and safety

Occupational Therapist: a form of therapy for those recuperating from physical or mental illness that encourages rehabilitation through the performance of activities required in daily life.

Ombudsman: one who speaks on behalf of another; a volunteer individual who helps residents in long-term care facilities

Omnibus Budget Reconciliation Act of 1987 (OBRA 87): The **Omnibus Reconciliation Act** of **1987** set forth new provisions for Medicare and Medicaid sections related to new standards for care in the nursing home setting. One major provision was for nurse aide training.

Open-ended question: question that requires a more complex answer than a simple "yes" or "no"

Organ: a part of an organism that is typically self-contained and has a specific vital function, such as the heart or liver in humans.

Organism: an individual animal, plant, or single-celled life form.

Organ System: The human body is the structure of a human being. It is composed of many different types of cells that together create tissues and subsequently organ systems. They ensure homeostasis and the viability of the human body.

Organize: arrange into a structured whole; order.

Orientation: level of awareness as to person, Place, and time

Orthosis: equipment or device, such as a brace or splint, used to provide support to a weak or injured part of the body

Orthostatic hypotension: a sudden drop in blood pressure associated with position change (lying to sitting or standing); resulting in fainting; inability of cardiovascular system to respond quickly enough to body position change, causing a drop-in blood pressure, often accompanied by dizziness, fainting or falls

Osteoarthritis: degenerative joint disease caused by wear and tear of the joint

orthopnea: difficulty breathing except when in an upright position

Orthopneic or Tripod Position: a position assumed to relieve orthopnea or difficulty breathing except when in the upright position; the patient assumes an upright or semi vertical position by using pillows to support the head and chest or sits upright in a chair.

Osteoporosis: a loss of minerals in the bones resulting in loss of bone density

Ostomy: surgical procedure that creates an opening from the intestine to outside the body for discharge of waste

Outbreak: sudden increase in cases of a disease within a certain geographic area or within a facility, school, community, etc.

Ovaries: glands in the female that produce ovum (eggs) and hormones

Overflow incontinence: associated with overdistention of the bladder caused by obstruction (e.g., enlarged prostate) or a neurological condition (e.g., spinal cord injury).

Oxygen: colorless, odorless reactive gas and a life-supporting component of the air.

Oxygen saturation: the percentage of hemoglobin binding sites in the bloodstream occupied by **oxygen**.

P

Pain: an unpleasant sensory and emotional experience associated with actual or potential tissue damage or described in terms of such damage

Palliative Care: care that focuses on providing comfort and improving quality of life by relieving pain and other symptoms particularly at end of life.

Pallor: paleness; a clinical manifestation consisting of an unnatural paleness of the skin.

Palpation: physical examination conducted by touching the resident's body with the fingers and/or hands

Paralanguage: component of communication by speech, for example intonation, pitch and speed of speaking, hesitation noises, gesture, and facial expression.

Paralyzed: absence of movement or sensation

Paranoia: suspiciousness inappropriate to reality; individual feels that everyone is picking on him/her or out to get him/her

Paranoid Disorders: personality disorders which involve odd or eccentric ways of thinking. People with PPD also suffer from paranoia, an unrelenting mistrust and suspicion of others, even when there is no reason to be suspicious

Paraplegia- paralysis of the legs

Parasite: organism that lives in or on another organism

Parkinson's Disease: neurological disease that affects motor skills

Passive range of motion exercises: movements the staff routinely conduct to prevent complication of immobility

Patience: Ability to remain calm even when the demands are heavy or seem unreasonable. The ability to endure waiting, delay, or provocation without becoming annoyed or upset, or to persevere calmly when faced with difficulties

Patient Self Determination Act of 1990 - requires hospitals, skilled nursing facilities, home health agencies, hospice programs, and health maintenance organizations to: (1) inform **patients** of their rights under State law to make decisions

Pathogens: microbes that cause disease

Percussion: tapping on a body area (chest, back, abdomen) to hear the sound that is produced; used to determine the status of internal organs and tissue

Periodontal Disease: an inflammatory **disease** that affects the soft and hard structures that support the teeth. In its early stage, called gingivitis, the gums become swollen and red due to inflammation, which is the body's natural response to the presence of harmful bacteria.

Perineal care: cleansing the genital and anal areas.

Perineal: the genital and anal areas

Peripheral vascular disease (PVD): condition that causes diminished blood flow to the extremities

Peristalsis: wavelike movements of the digestive tract that move food through the intestinal tract

Peritoneal Dialysis: type of dialysis in which waste and fluid are removed from the body using a surgically placed catheter in the abdominal (peritoneal) cavity

Perpetrator: person who inflicts harm

Personal care: care provided for residents that includes bathing, mouth care, hair care, grooming and dressing

Person-centered care: "Providing care that is respectful of, and responsive to, individual patient preferences, needs and values, and ensuring that patient values guide all clinical decisions."

Personal health record (PHR): A **personal health record** (**PHR**) is a health record where health data and other information related to the care of a patient is maintained by the patient. The intention of a PHR is to provide a complete and accurate summary of an individual's medical history which is accessible online. The health data on a PHR might include patient-reported outcome data, lab results, and data from devices such as wireless electronic weighing scales or (collected passively).

Personality: the combination of characteristics or qualities that form an individual's distinctive character.

Pharmacological: relating to the branch of medicine concerned with the uses, effects, and modes of action of drugs. When discussing interventions, a pharmacological approach would include the use of medications.

Pharynx: the throat

Physical: relating to the body and bodily functions

Physical Abuse: "Physical abuse" includes hitting, slapping, punching and kicking. It also includes controlling behavior through corporal punishment.

Physical Therapist: a form of therapy that maintains or improves physical abilities (posture, walking, Range of Motion). The treatment of disease, injury, or deformity by physical methods such as massage, heat treatment, and exercise rather than by drugs or surgery

Physical restraint: any manual method or physical or manual device, material, or equipment attached or adjacent to the resident's body that the individual cannot remove easily and that restricts freedom of movement or normal access to one's body

Physiologic: Characteristic of normal, healthy functioning of a living organism.

Plan of Correction: the response to the SOD in which the facility surveyed states how it will correct the deficiencies identified by the State survey agency. CMS defines a Plan of Correction to mean a plan developed by the facility and approved by CMS or the survey agency that describes the actions the facility will take to correct deficiencies and specifies the date by which those deficiencies will be corrected.

Plaque: sticky, transparent bacterial film found on the teeth

Pleural Effusion: excess fluid that accumulates in the pleural cavity, the fluid-filled space that surrounds the lungs

Pneumonia: inflammation of the lungs with fluid accumulation in the acted alveoli

Podiatrist: physician speciating in the care and treatment of the feet

Policy and Procedure (P&P): guidelines and procedures established by the facility for daily operations and emergency/disaster situations

Political: relating to the government or the public affairs of a country.

Portal of Entry: opening by which a microorganism enters a host

Portal of Exit: the place a microorganism leaves the reservoir

Positioning: assisting a resident in changing position

Position change alarms are alerting devices intended to monitor a resident's movement. The devices emit an audible signal when the resident moves in certain ways.

Positive Attitude: Sense of enjoying your job and ability to integrate the good character qualities into your work, accepting job assignments in a positive manner.

Post-acute care unit: unit that provides a high level of care for residents including rehabilitation units

Posterior: toward the back, back of the body

Position: a certain arrangement of bodily parts

Postmortem: after death

Post-operative: period of time after surgery

Post-Traumatic Stress Disorder (PTSD): Involves the development of symptoms following exposure to one or more traumatic, life-threatening events

Posture: the position or bearing of the body whether characteristi c or assumed for a special purpose

Precipitating Factors: associated with the definitive onset of a disease, illness, accident, behavioral response, or course of action. (resident was changing from bed to standing c/o dizziness and fell-precipitating factor was position change)

Preferences: The view that one person, object, or course of action is more desirable than another, or a choice based on such a view, the right or opportunity to choose a person, object, or course of action that is considered more desirable than another. *In social models of care allowing resident preference to dictate schedules and daily choices such as dressing, time to get up, time to go to bed, etc.*

Preoperative: period of time before surgery

Presbyopia: Age-related hearing loss. It is the loss of hearing that gradually occurs in most of us as we grow older. It is one of the most common conditions affecting older and elderly adults.

Pressure Ulcer: an ulcer that forms on the skin over a bony area as a result of pressure

Primary Site: the first organ or body system affected by cancer

Priorities or Priority: should be done first; the state of having most importance or urgency, somebody or something that is ranked highly in terms of importance or urgency. *"Things that matter the least must never be at the mercy of things that matter the most."*

Privileged Communication: any personal or private information that is relevant to a resident's care that the resident gave to medical personnel

Procrastinating: delay or postpone action; put off doing something

Productive Cough: raising mucus or sputum (as from the bronchi)

Professional: Conforming to the standards of skill, competence, or character normally expected of a properly qualified and experienced person in a work environment. *The CNA dresses professionally and demonstrates a high degree of professional character.*

Professionalism: the competence or skill expected of a professional or the conduct, aims, or qualities that characterize or mark a profession or a professional person

Projectile Vomiting: vomitus forcibly ejected without nausea

Pronation: to turn downward

Prone Position: lying on the belly

Prostate cancer: cancer of the prostate gland in males

Protective Oversight: an awareness twenty-four hours a day of the location of a resident, the ability to intervene on behalf of the resident, the supervision of nutrition, medication, or actual provisions of care, and the responsibility for the welfare of the resident, except where the resident is on voluntary leave.

Prosthesis: an artificial body part

Protein: large molecules composed of one or more long chains of amino acids and are an essential part of all living organisms, especially as structural components of body tissues such as muscle, hair, collagen, etc., and as enzymes and antibodies. A substance that has amino acids, compounds and carbon, hydrogen, oxygen, nitrogen and sometimes sulfur and is found in many foods.

Protocol: official or standard way of doing something usually put in writing

Proximal - Center of the Body

Psychological: associated with the thought processes of the brain,

Psychosocial: relating to psychological and social aspects of mental health

Psychosocial needs: the mental needs that motivate a person to achieve goals and perform certain activities

Pulse: the beat of the heart felt at an artery as a wave of blood passes through the artery

Pulse rate: the number of heartbeats or pulses felt in 1 minute

Pulse oximeter: monitoring a person's oxygen saturation

Purulent: containing pus

Pus: thick yellowish secretion formed in certain kinds of inflammation

Q

Quadriplegia: paralysis of the arms and legs

Quality Indicator Survey (QIS): process for annual evaluation of facility quality of care directed by state/federal survey system

Quality of life: how good or bad a person's life is from their own perspective.

R

RACE: Fire acronym R-Rescue, A=Activate, C=Contain and E=Extinguish

Radial Pulse: pulse measurement taken by feeling the pulse at the radial artery at the wrist

Radiation therapy: treatment for cancer or other disease using x-ray or other forms of radiation

Range of motion (ROM): the extent of movement of a joint (maximum flexion and maximum extension)

Rash: an eruption on the body

Reality Orientation: technique used to assist a person to become aware of the world in which he/she lives (used much less frequently with dementia then it used to be)

Rectum: last 6-8 inches of the rectum

Reflection: restating in your own words what another person has said to be sure that you understand the speakers meaning and feelings

Registered Dietician (RD): staff member who develops food plans and special diets for residents

Registered Nurse: An individual who has graduated from a state-approved school of nursing, passed the NCLEX-RN Examination and is licensed by a state board of nursing to provide patient care.

Regulatory Survey: Survey of long-term care facility every 9 to 15 months whereby all areas of care and services are reviewed at the long-term care facility.

Regulated waste: contaminated waste that must be disposed of according to facility policies and government regulations

Rehabilitation: restoring of an ill or injured patient so he/she will be able to help himself/herself to live at his/her maximum or highest potential

Reliable: consistently good in quality or performance; able to be trusted, a person or thing with trustworthy qualities

Reliability: Taking ownership of your job; dependability; ability to perform duties without fail; being on time for work and following policy and procedures for calling in absent. Able to be trusted to do what is expected or has been promised, able to be trusted to be accurate or to provide a correct result

Relocation stress syndrome: stress and anxiety experienced by a person relocating to a new environment, such as a resident entering a nursing home

"**Removes easily**" the manual method, physical or mechanical device, equipment, or material, can be removed intentionally by the resident in the same manner as it was applied by the staff.

Report: To give information about something that has happened to give detailed information about a resident or policy changes at the facility.

Reproductive System: body system made up of reproductive organs and glands

Resident: A person who, due to aging or illness, receives or requires care and the services furnished by a facility and who lives at the facility.

Residential Care Facility (RCF) I or II: A facility licensed by the state of Missouri to provide 24-hour room, board, and protective oversight. The facility may provide assistance with medications, care during recovery from short-term illness, supervision of diets, and assistance with personal care.

Resident Rights The resident has a right to a dignified existence, self-determination, and communication with and access to persons and services inside and outside the facility. All residents in long term care facilities have rights guaranteed to them under Federal and State law.

Residue: what remains of something after a part is removed

Resistance: ability to fight off

Resistance to care: reluctance or refusal to participate or allow care to be provided

Reservoir: person, animal or environment in which an infectious agent lives

Resident Assessment Instrument (RAI): assessment tool used in long term care facilities to document key information about residents, including care plans and outcomes. The MDS is a part of this assessment process.

Resident Council: an organization of people living together in a common place. Similar to a tenants' association, councils represent the interests of those living together and provide a way for residents to have a say in the way their home is run

Respect: A feeling or attitude of admiration and deference toward somebody or something, consideration, or thoughtfulness.

Respiration: act of breathing in and out of the lungs (inhalation/exhalation)

Respiration rate: measurement of the number of breaths per minute

Respiratory System: body system that allows for the exchange of oxygen and carbon dioxide in the body

Respite care: care provided for residents who enter a facility for a temporary stay

Responsibility: The state, fact, or position of being accountable to somebody or for something. Earning authority to make decisions independently which are appropriate for the CNA.

"Acknowledge and respect the rights of others. Cultivate the habit of doing our duties at all times and performing at our best, no matter how we feel.

Responsible Party: a family member/friend of the resident who the resident designates in writing to handle matters and receive reports related to the resident's general condition.

Restraint: a measure/ device or condition that keeps someone or something under control or within limits

Retribution: punishment inflicted on someone as vengeance for a wrong or criminal act.

Restorative Nurse Assistant (RNA): A CNA who has received additional training in restorative nursing procedures (mobility, range of motion, positioning, etc.) who works under the supervision of a registered nurse or licensed nurse to assist with restorative nursing practices.

Routine: The usual sequence for a set of activities, regular or standard and not out of the ordinary. *Allowing time and respect for the resident's routines, preferences and history, such as when they get up, how they do morning grooming, when they bath and how often.*

Restorative: returning a resident to health or consciousness

Restorative nursing: the process by which a disabled or ill person is helped to reach the highest possible level of wellness, considering his/her limitations

Retention: inability to empty the bladder

Rheumatoid arthritis: autoimmune disease that causes inflammation of the joints

Rhythm: a characteristic rhythmic pattern

Routine care: daily care activities

Rights: Rights are legal, social, or ethical principles of freedom or entitlement; that is, rights are the fundamental normative rules about what is allowed of people or owed to people, according to some legal system, social convention, or ethical theory. They are things we are entitled to by law, norms of society, etc.

Rigor Mortis: temporary rigidity of muscles of the body occurring after death

Rheumatoid Arthritis: is a long-term autoimmune disorder that primarily affects joints. It typically results in warm, swollen, and painful joints

Rotation: to move a joint in a circular motion

Roughage/Fiber: indigestible fiber of fruits, vegetables, and cereal that acts as a stimulus to aid intestinal peristalsis (e.g., bran, potato skins, fruit skins)

S

Safety data sheet (SDS) or material safety data sheet (MSDS), or product safety data sheet (PSDS): documents that list information relating to occupational safety and health for the use of various substances and products.

Sarcopenia: loss of muscle tissue as a natural part of the aging process

Schizophrenia: is a chronic brain disorder that affects less than one percent of the U.S. population. When schizophrenia is active, symptoms can include delusions, hallucinations, trouble with thinking and concentration, and lack of motivation.

Scope: the extent of the area or subject matter that something deals with or to which it is relevant. There are three levels that are used to determine the scope of a deficiency: isolated, pattern, or widespread. The scope levels reflect how many residents were affected by the deficiencies cited and are described below:

- Isolated: When one or a very limited number of residents or employees is/are affected and/or a very limited area or number of locations within the facility are affected;
- Pattern: When more than a very limited number of residents or employees are affected, and/or the situation has occurred in more than a limited number of locations, but the locations are not dispersed throughout the facility;
- Widespread: When the problems causing the deficiency are pervasive (affect many locations) throughout the facility and/or represent a systemic failure that affected, or has the potential to affect, a large portion or all of the residents or employees.

Scrotum: the pouch containing the testicles

Secretions: substances such as saliva, mucus, perspiration, tears, etc. that come out of the body

Sebaceous glands: microscopic glands in the skin that secrete an oily substance called sebum

Seizure: a sudden, periodic attacks of muscles contracting and relaxing

Self-Actualization: the realization or fulfillment of one's talents and potentialities, especially considered as a drive or need present in everyone.

Self-care: the practice of taking action to preserve or improve one's own health and caring for one’s own needs.

Self-Confidence: Confidence in yourself and your own abilities

Self-Determination: the process by which a person determines his or her own care, life choices, etc. with freedom and independence to do so.

Self-Discovery: the process of acquiring insight into one's own character.

Self-esteem: Confidence in your own merit as an individual person

Self-mastery: Having inner virtues, such as control over your impulses. A complete and individual personality, especially one that somebody recognizes as his or her own and with which there is a sense of ease. *"The resident was very angry and said some hurtful things. The CNA remained outwardly calm and dignified while continuing to provide care."" Live courteously and use good manners toward everyone without exception and do this even in the face of rudeness or provocation.*

Self-worth: the sense of one's own value or worth as a person.

Senses: vision, hearing, equilibrium (balance), smell, taste, touch

Sensitivity: Awareness of attitudes and feelings of others; knowing when a person feels uncomfortable, lonely, scared, etc.; awareness of a cultural diversity and unique resident needs. Care and understanding of needs and requirements, capacity for physical sensation or response. "*The CNA was sensitive to Mrs. J's feelings today. She just learned that her daughter passed away.*"

Service mentality: dedication to making sure that customers' needs are satisfied

Serous - Thin and Watery

Severity: There are four factors that determine the severity (degree of harm or potential harm) of a deficiency:

- Level 1 - No actual harm with potential for minimal harm: A deficiency that has the potential for causing no more than a minor negative impact on the residents or employees;
- Level 2 - No actual harm with a potential for more than minimal harm that is not immediate jeopardy: Noncompliance with the requirements that results in the potential for no more than minimal physical, mental, and/or psychosocial harm to the residents or employees and/or that result in minimal discomfort to the residents or employees of the facility, but has the potential to result in more than minimal harm that is not immediate jeopardy;
- Level 3 - Actual harm that is not immediate jeopardy: Noncompliance with the requirements that results in actual harm to residents or employees that is not immediate jeopardy;
- Level 4 - Immediate jeopardy to resident health or safety: Noncompliance with the requirements that results in immediate jeopardy to resident or employee health or safety in

which immediate corrective action is necessary because the provider's noncompliance with one or more of those requirements has caused, or is likely to cause, serious injury, harm, impairment, or death to a resident receiving care in a facility or an employee of the facility.

Sexual Abuse: Includes, but is not limited to, sexual harassment, sexual coercion, or sexual assault. Sexual abuse is non-consensual sexual contact of any type with a resident.

Sexual Activity: Includes sexual contact and other activities intended to cause sexual arousal (e.g. viewing sexually explicit photographs and videos, reading sexually explicit text, and phone sex.)

Sexual Contact: Includes sexual intercourse, oral sex, masturbation, and sexual touch.

Sexually transmitted disease (STD): infectious disease transmitted through sexual contact

Sharp: adapted to cutting or piercing

Shearing: occurs when the body slides on a surface that moves the skin in one direction and the underlying bone in the opposite direction (can cause tissue damage)

Shock: medical emergency in which body tissues and organs are not receiving enough oxygen and blood

Shortness of Breath: difficulty breathing

Shuffling: to move by sliding along or back and forth without lifting

Significant change of Condition: a major decline or improvement in a resident's status that:

1. Will not normally resolve itself without intervention by staff or by implementing standard disease-related clinical interventions, the decline is not considered "self- limiting".
2. Impacts more than one area of the resident's health status: and
3. Requires interdisciplinary review and/or revision of the care plan.

Signs: an object, quality, or event whose presence or occurrence indicates the probable presence or occurrence of something else. *Blood coming out a nostril is a sign; it is apparent to the patient, physician, and others.*

Sitz bath: bath in a tub or special basin in which only the perineum and buttocks are immersed

Skilled nursing facility (SNF): A facility that provides 24-hour room, board, and skilled nursing care and treatment to at least three residents. Skilled nursing care and treatment services are those performed by or under the supervision of a registered nurse for individuals requiring 24-hour-a-day care by licensed nursing personnel and under the direction of a licensed nurse.

Slander: to make oral defamatory false remarks about another, spoken words that tend to damage the reputation of another

Social: relating to human society, getting along with others

Social model of care: Means long-term care services based on the abilities, desires, and functional needs of the individual delivered in a setting that is more home-like than institutional, that promote the dignity, individuality, privacy, independence, and autonomy of the individual, that respects residents' differences and promotes residents' choices.

Social Service Designee: social service representative appointed to take care of certain responsibilities (a facility position)

Spasm: an involuntary and abnormal muscular contraction

Specimen: sample of fluid or tissue taken for examination and/or testing

Sputum: mixture of saliva and mucus coughed up from the respiratory tract, typically as a result of infection or other disease and often examined microscopically to aid medical diagnosis.

Speech Therapy: A discipline of therapy involved in the evaluation, diagnosis, and treatment of communication disorders (speech disorders and language disorders), cognitive-communication disorders, voice disorders, and swallowing disorders

Speech Therapist: therapist who work with speech, and other communication disorders as well as with swallowing disorders to improve speech, language or swallowing abilities.

Splint: device used to support or immobilize a body part

Sphincter muscles: a circle of muscle fibers around the outlet of the urethra and rectum that is normally closed but can be relaxed to allow passage of urine or stool

Sphygmomanometer: instrument used to measure BP that consists of a cuff that is applied to the upper arm and a measuring device

Spiritual Counselor: Coordinates religious services and provides counseling for residents and families.

Spiritual distress, the feeling that the future is hopeless

Spirituality is defined as finding the inner meaning, or essence of life.

Sputum: waste material coughed up from lungs or trachea

Standard precautions: evidence-based practices designed to prevent transmission of infectious disease

Statement of Deficiencies (SOD): After the State survey agency completes its survey, it sends the entity surveyed a statement of deficiencies which is a document that communicates to the provider or supplier (Facility) surveyed what is wrong and forms the basis for the plan of correction that the entity surveyed provides to the State survey agency. The Statement of Deficiencies, form CMS-2567 is the official documentation to record deficiencies

State Operations Manual (SOM) : The manual that outlines the procedures, regulations with interpretative guidance and required forms for Long Term Care (LTC) facilities and is the surveyors guide to the survey processes required by CMS.

Steady: direct or sure in movement, firm in position

Sterile: free of all germs

Sterilization: process that eliminates all microorganisms from a surface or object

Stethoscope: instrument used to listen to the sounds produced by the heart, lungs, and other body organs

Stimuli: something that rouses or incites to activity

Stoma: surgically created opening that is kept open for drainage or the removal of waste

Strategy: a plan or method

Stress: a state of mental or emotional strain or tension resulting from adverse or very demanding circumstances

Stress Incontinence: a condition (found chiefly in women) in which there is involuntary emission of urine when pressure within the abdomen increases suddenly, as in coughing or jumping.

Subclinical: relating to or denoting a disease which is not severe enough to present definite or readily observable symptoms.

Subcutaneous: under the skin

Subjective information: information based on an assumption, opinion, or on what the resident says about how they feel

Substance Abuse and Addiction: a medical condition in which the use of one or more substances leads to a clinically significant impairment or distress.

Substandard Quality of Care (SQOC): a technical regulatory term which means that one or more requirements under the federal regulations 42CFR 483.13 (resident behavior and facility practices), 42CFR 483.15 (quality of life), or 42CFR 483.25 (quality of care) were not met, to a degree constituting immediate jeopardy to resident health or safety, and a scope of pattern or widespread actual harm, or a widespread potential for more than minimal harm. A finding of substandard quality of care indicates that the nursing home was found to have had a significant deficiency (or deficiencies), which the home must address and correct quickly to protect the health and safety of residents.

Sundowning: phenomenon when confusion becomes worse in the evening

Supination: to turn upward

Supine: lying on one's back

Suppository: a semisolid substance that may contain medicine that dissolves when inserted into the rectum or vagina

Susceptible host: Any person, the most vulnerable of whom are receiving care, are immunocompromised or have invasive medical devices. A member of a population who is at risk of becoming infected by a disease

Suprapubic Catheter: hollow flexible tube that is used to drain urine from the bladder. It is inserted into the bladder through a cut in abdominal wall, a few inches below the navel.

Survey: is an information-gathering process and is conducted by state-level personnel who review facility processes for compliance with state and federal requirements that all long-term care facilities who accept Medicare or Medicaid residents are subject to.

Susceptible host: a person who is at risk for developing an infection from a microorganism

Symptoms: subjective evidence of disease. *Anxiety, low back pain, and fatigue are all* ***symptoms****; only the patient can perceive them.*

Systemic: effecting the whole body

Systolic Pressure: amount of force it takes to pump blood out of the heart into the arterial circulation (the top number when measuring B/P)

T

Tachycardia: fast pulse rate greater than 100 beats per minute

TED hose: elastic stockings applies to the legs to reduce inflammation of the veins and the formation of blood clots

Temperature: measurement of heat within the body

Terminal condition: illnesses from which a patient is not expected to recover; death will likely occur within a short period of time

Terminal disinfection: thorough cleaning of room with disinfectant solution after transmission-based procedure is discontinued

Testes: two oval glands that produce sperm cells and secrete male sex hormones; also called testicles

Therapeutic: referring to a treatment

Therapeutic diet: special diet used as a treatment for a disease or condition

Time Management: To plan the moment or occasion for something, especially in order to achieve the best result or effect. *Use your time properly and effectively in a manner that allows ample time for getting your duties done in a timely manner.*

Tissue: any of the distinct types of material of which animals or plants are made, consisting of specialized cells and their products.

Tolerance: capacity to endure pain or hardship

Total parenteral nutrition (TPN): nutrition administered intravenously

Toxin: a poisonous substance

Tracheostomy: creation of an opening into the trachea to facilitate breathing; also known as tracheotomy

Transfer: to move

Transient ischemic attack (TIA): an episode of poor circulation to the brain characterized by visual disturbances, dizziness, weakness, numbness, or loss of consciousness. The attack is usually brief, lasting only a few minutes

Transmitted: (transfer or spread), passed on from one person or place to another.

Trapeze: suspended horizontal bar used to help position a person in bed

Trauma: a deeply distressing or disturbing experience or a physical injury

Tremors: a trembling or shaking usually from physical weakness, emotional stress, or disease

Trendelenburg Position - Lying Face-Up with Feet Elevated

Triggers: A trigger is something that sets off a memory, flashback or behavior. In trauma it may transport the person back to the event of her/his original trauma. Triggers are very personal; different things trigger different people.

Tuberculosis: an infection, primarily of the lung, from mycobacterium tuberculosis

Turning and Repositioning: Place in a different position. Proper turning and repositioning is a method to reduce the chance of tissue breakdown and wound development.

Twenty-Four Hour Clock: The **24-hour clock** is the convention of **time** keeping in which the day runs from midnight to midnight and is divided into **24 hours**, indicated by the **hours** passed since midnight, from 0 to 23.

U

Uncomplicated Nursing Procedures: Are non-invasive procedures that do not require licensed nurses to perform directly, such as measuring vital signs, providing personal hygiene, etc..

Unconscious: an individual's lacking in awareness

Unsteady: not firm or solid: not fixed in position

Ureters: tubes that carry urine from kidneys to urinary bladder

Urethra: the small passage from the bladder through which urine leaves the body

Urge incontinence: involuntary leakage accompanied or immediately proceeded by urgency

Urgent: requiring immediate action or attention.

Urinalysis: physical, chemical, and microscopic examination of a urine sample

Urinary catheter: a sterile tube inserted into bladder to drain urine

Urinary System: body system that helps maintain fluid balance and eliminates liquid waste

Urinary Tract Infection (UTI): an infection that affects part of the urinary tract. When it affects the lower urinary tract, it is known as a bladder infection (cystitis) and when it affects the upper urinary tract it is known as a kidney infection (pyelonephritis)

Urinary Output: amount of urine produced and expelled

Urinate (void): to pass urine

Urine: liquid waste produced by the kidneys and stored in the bladder

V

Vaccine: a substance used to stimulate the production of antibodies and provide immunity against one or several diseases, prepared from the causative agent of a disease, its products, or a synthetic substitute, treated to act as an antigen without inducing the disease.

Validation therapy: a technique that creates a climate of acceptance by encouraging the resident who is confused to explore personal thoughts, it helps to confirm the emotions being experienced

Value System: behavior related to a pattern of conduct or ideas that is accepted as worthwhile or meaningful

Vector: living agent that transmits infection

Vehicle: some type of inanimate object that acts as a carrier for microorganism

Vein: blood vessels that carry deoxygenated blood from the body back to the heart and lungs

Ventilate: give air to

Verbal Abuse: The use of oral, written, or gestured language that willfully includes disparaging and derogatory terms to residents or their families, or within their hearing distance, regardless of their age, ability to comprehend, or disability. Examples of verbal abuse include, but are not limited to threats of harm; saying things to frighten a resident, such as telling a resident that he/she will never be able to see his/her family again.

Verbal communication: sending and receiving messages using spoken or written words

Virtue: The quality of being morally good or righteous. "*To do something with good grace when you are obligated to do it anyway. To stay committed to what you know and learn to be right when caring for residents. Positive virtues for the CNA as well as the organization include trust, encouragement, mutual respect, cooperation, collaboration and selflessness.*"

Virus: a type of microorganism that survives only in living things

Vital signs: temperature, pulse, respirations, and blood pressure

Vitamin: an organic substance found in foods and essential in small quantities for growth, health, and the preservation of life itself. The body needs vitamins just as it requires other food constituents such as proteins, fats, carbohydrates, minerals, and water. ... Vitamins serve as coenzymes or cofactors in enzymatic reactions.

Void: to empty the bladder; urinate

Volition: A resident's clear, unequivocal, unforced willing participation in an intimate relationship or sexual activity. Freedom from coercion is a trait of volition. In this document "Consenting resident" means a resident whose participation in an intimate relationship or sexual activity is volitional.

W

Walking Rounds: In some facilities the CNA's and charge nurse conduct walking rounds. Going down the halls to each person's room and reporting on any new or unusual circumstances for that resident.

Wandering: aimless walking, which may result in a resident becoming lost

Well-being: the state of being comfortable, healthy, or happy.

Wheezing: to breathe with difficulty usually with a whistling sound

Willful: acting deliberately

Willingness: Eager to learn and help others.; Working as part of the health care team. Ready to do something without being forced cooperative and enthusiastic

Wisdom: Exerting sound judgment, the ability to make sensible decisions and judgments based on personal knowledge and experience, good sense shown in a way of thinking, judgment, or action, accumulated knowledge of life or of a sphere of activity that has been gained through experience

X

Xerostomia: dryness in the mouth, which may be associated with a change in the composition of saliva, or reduced salivary flow, or have no identifiable cause

Appendix B

Common Medical Abbreviations

a: before

a.c.: before meals

Abd: abdomen

ad lib: at will, as desired

ADL: Activity of Daily Living

adm: admission, admitted

AM: Morning

amb: ambulate

amt: amount

AP: apical

ASAP: as soon as possible

bid: twice a day

BM: bowel movement

B/P or BP: blood pressure

BR: Bedrest

BRP: bathroom privileges

BSC: Bedside Commode

c: with

cath: catheter

cap: capsule

cc: cubic centimeter

c/o: complains of

C02: carbon dioxide

CPR: cardiopulmonary resuscitation

CVA: cerebrovascular accident: stroke

CXR: chest x-ray

d/c: discontinue or discharge

DON: Director of Nursing

Drsg or dsg: dressing

dx: diagnosis

ECG or EKG: electrocardiogram

EBL: estimated blood loss

ER: emergency room

F: Fahrenheit

FF: Force fluids

ft. foot

fb: foreign body

fx: fracture

gtt: drop-liquid measurement

h or hr: hour

H2O: water

HA: Headache

HOH: Hard of hearing

H & P: history and physical

HR: heart rate

hs: hour of sleep (bedtime)

ht: height

i: 1

ii: 2

iii: 3

iv: 4

v: 5

I & O: intake and output

ICP: Intradisciplinary care plan

IDDM: insulin dependent diabetes mellitus

IV: intravenous

IM: intramuscular

kg: kilogram (2.2 kg=1 lb)

l or lt: left

MD: medical doctor

Mg: milligram

midnoc: midnight

ml: milliliter

NA: Sodium

NAS: no added salt

neg: negative

NPO: nothing by mouth

noc: night

O2: oxygen

OD: right eye

OS: left eye

OU: both eyes

OOB: Out of bed

OT: occupational therapy

p̄: after

PM: Afternoon or evening

po: by mouth

PR: Per rectum

post-op: postoperative (after surgery)

pre-op: preoperative (before surgery)

pt: patient

prn: as needed

pc: after meals

PT: Physical Therapy

q: every

qd: every day

qh: every hour

qhs: every hour of sleep

qid: four times a day

qod: every other day

q2h, q3h, q4h, etc.: every 2 hours, every 3 hours, every 4 hours, etc.

R or rt: right

RCP: Resident care plan

res: resident

ROM: Range of Motion

RX: prescription, treatment

sc/sq: subcutaneous

s: without

sx: symptoms

s/s: signs and symptoms

stat: immediately

SOB: short of breath

spec: specimen

tab: tablet

tid: three times a day

TPR: temperature, pulse, respiration

UA: urinalysis

vs: vital signs

W/C: wheelchair

wt: weight

x: times

Appendix C

Common Medical Diagnosis for Elderly

Alzheimer's Disease: progressive mental deterioration that can occur in middle or old age, due to generalized degeneration of the brain. It is the most common cause of premature senility. **Amyotrophic Lateral Sclerosis (ALS):** Amyotrophic lateral sclerosis (ALS), also known as motor neuron disease (MND) or Lou Gehrig's disease, is a specific disease that causes the death of neurons controlling voluntary muscles

Arrhythmia of the Heart: a condition in which the heart beats with an irregular or abnormal rhythm.

Arthritis: painful inflammation and stiffness of the joints.

Atrial Fibrillation: is an abnormal heart rhythm characterized by rapid and irregular beating of the atrial chambers of the heart. Often it starts as brief periods of abnormal beating which become longer and possibly constant over time

Autism: a developmental disorder of variable severity that is characterized by difficulty in social interaction and communication and by restricted or repetitive patterns of thought and behavior

Decubitus Ulcers or Pressure Ulcers: localized damage to the skin and/or underlying tissue that usually occur over a bony prominence as a result of usually long-term pressure, or pressure in combination with shear or friction. The most common sites are the skin overlying the sacrum, coccyx, heels, and hips, though other sites can be affected, such as the elbows, knees, ankles, back of shoulders, or the back of the cranium.

Bipolar Disorder (Manic-depressive illness): a mental disorder that causes periods of depression and abnormally elevated moods

Cancer: a group of diseases involving abnormal cell growth with the potential to invade or spread to other parts of the body

Cataracts: A cataract is a clouding of the lens in the eye which leads to a decrease in vision.

Chronic Kidney Failure: a type of kidney disease in which there is gradual loss of kidney function over a period of months to years. Initially there are generally no symptoms; later, symptoms may include leg swelling, feeling tired, vomiting, loss of appetite, and confusion.

COPD, or Chronic Obstructive Pulmonary Disease: a type of obstructive lung disease characterized by long-term breathing problems and poor airflow.

Diabetes: a disease in which the body's ability to produce or respond to the hormone insulin is impaired, resulting in abnormal metabolism of carbohydrates and elevated levels of glucose in the blood and urine.

Fibromyalgia: a chronic disorder characterized by widespread musculoskeletal pain, fatigue, and tenderness in localized areas.

Glaucoma: a condition of increased pressure within the eyeball, causing gradual loss of sight.

Heart Disease: a range of conditions that affect the heart. Diseases under the heart disease umbrella include blood vessel diseases, such as coronary artery disease; heart rhythm problems (arrhythmias); and heart defects

Hepatitis: a disease characterized by inflammation of the liver.

HIV/AIDS: human immunodeficiency virus, a retrovirus which causes AIDS.

Hypertension (High Blood Pressure): abnormally high blood pressure

Hyperthyroidism (overactive thyroid): overactivity of the thyroid gland, resulting in a rapid heartbeat and an increased rate of metabolism.

Hypothyroidism (underactive thyroid): abnormally low activity of the thyroid gland, resulting in retardation of growth and mental development in children and adults

Irritable Bowel Syndrome (IBS): a group of symptoms—including abdominal pain and changes in the pattern of bowel movements without any evidence of underlying damage.

Inflammatory Bowel Disease (IBD): a group of inflammatory conditions of the colon and small intestine. Crohn's disease and ulcerative colitis are the principal types of inflammatory bowel disease

Kidney Failure, Chronic: also known as end-stage kidney disease, is a medical condition in which the kidneys are functioning at less than 15% of normal. Kidney failure is classified as either acute kidney failure, which develops rapidly and may resolve; and chronic kidney failure, which develops slowly

Leukemia: a malignant progressive disease in which the bone marrow and other blood-forming organs produce increased numbers of immature or abnormal leukocytes. These suppress the production of normal blood cells, leading to anemia and other symptoms.

Liver Failure, Acute: the appearance of severe complications rapidly after the first signs of liver disease (such as jaundice) and indicates that the liver has sustained severe damage (loss of function of 80–90% of liver cells).

Lupus: a systemic autoimmune disease that occurs when the body's immune system attacks its own tissues and organs. Inflammation caused by lupus can affect many different body systems — including joints, skin, kidneys, blood cells, brain, heart and lungs.

Lymphoma, Hodgkin's (Hodgkin's disease): a type of lymphoma in which cancer originates from a specific type of white blood cells called lymphocytes.

Lymphoma, Non-Hodgkin's: a group of blood cancers that includes all types of lymphoma except Hodgkin's lymphomas

Macular Degeneration, Dry: age-related macular degeneration (AMD or ARMD), is a medical condition which may result in blurred or no vision in the center of the visual field

Melanoma, Skin Cancer: a tumor of melanin-forming cells, especially a malignant tumor associated with skin cancer.

Multiple Sclerosis (MS): a disease in which the insulating covers of nerve cells in the brain and spinal cord are damaged. This damage disrupts the ability of parts of the nervous system to communicate, resulting in a range of signs and symptoms, including physical, mental, and sometimes psychiatric problems

Obstructive Sleep Apnea: A sleep disorder that is marked by pauses in breathing of 10 seconds or more during sleep and causes unrestful sleep.

Osteoarthritis: degeneration of joint cartilage and the underlying bone, most common from middle age onward. It causes pain and stiffness, especially in the hip, knee, and thumb joints.

Osteoporosis: a medical condition in which the bones become brittle and fragile from loss of tissue, typically because of hormonal changes, or deficiency of calcium or vitamin D.

Pancreatic Cancer: arises when cells in the pancreas, a glandular organ behind the stomach, begin to multiply out of control and form a mass. These cancerous cells have the ability to invade other parts of the body.

Parkinson's Disease: a long-term degenerative disorder of the central nervous system that mainly affects the motor system

Periodontitis: inflammation of the tissue around the teeth, often causing shrinkage of the gums and loosening of the teeth.

Pneumonia: lung inflammation caused by bacterial or viral infection, in which the air sacs fill with pus and may become solid. Inflammation may affect both lungs (double pneumonia), one lung (single pneumonia), or only certain lobes (lobar pneumonia).

Post-traumatic stress disorder (PTSD): a mental disorder that can develop after a person is exposed to a traumatic event, such as sexual assault, warfare, traffic collisions, child abuse, or other threats on a person's life. Symptoms may include disturbing thoughts, feelings, or dreams related to the events, mental or physical distress to trauma-related cues, attempts to avoid trauma-related cues, alterations in how a person thinks and feels, and an increase in the fight-or-flight response

Rheumatoid Arthritis: a long-term autoimmune disorder that primarily affects joints. It typically results in warm, swollen, and painful joints.

Staph Infections: an infection caused by members of the Staphylococcus genus of bacteria. These bacteria commonly inhabit the skin and nose where they are innocuous but may enter the body through cuts or abrasions which may be nearly invisible. Once inside the body, the bacterium may spread to several body systems and organs

Stroke: a medical condition in which poor blood flow to the brain results in cell death.

Thrush, Oral: infection of the mouth and throat by a yeast like fungus, causing whitish patches. Also called candidiasis.

Transient Ischemic Attack (TIA): a brief episode of neurological dysfunction caused by loss of blood flow in the brain, spinal cord, or retina, without tissue death

Tuberculosis (TB): an infectious bacterial disease characterized by the growth of nodules (tubercles) in the tissues, especially the lungs

Ulcerative Colitis: a long-term condition that results in inflammation and ulcers of the colon and rectum.

Vascular Dementia: dementia caused by problems in the supply of blood to the brain, typically a series of minor strokes, leading to worsening cognitive decline that occurs step by step

Vertigo: a sensation of whirling and loss of balance, associated particularly with looking down from a great height, or caused by disease affecting the inner ear or the vestibular nerve; giddiness

Unit I Lesson Plan 1 Workbook Exercises

<u>Unit I LP 1: A. Person-Centered Care "Putting a Face on those you care for</u>:

Select a resident or patient that you would like to get to know. Go to them, introduce yourself and explain that you have an assignment on helping you to become a better CNA. Set down, establish eye contact, and ask them to tell you about themselves. If their hesitant, ask some open-ended questions? Here is a list of possible questions. Jot the answers down and then convert it to a story. Do not put a name on it and post it where other staff can see it. Can they figure out who it is about?

- Where did you grow up?
- Do you have a favorite memory of your parents?
- Did you have any brothers or sisters?
- What is a favorite memory of your childhood?
- Did you marry?
- Tell me about your spouse?
- What is a favorite memory of your spouse?
- Did you have children?
- How many and were they boys or girls?
- What is a favorite memory of raising your kids?
- What did you do for a living?
- Tell me about how that impacted your life?
- What is one thing you would like me to know about you when caring for you that would make you happy?
- Tell me about getting ready for bed at night?
- What was your routine?
-

Unit I LP 2 Workbook Exercises

<u>Unit I LP 1. B. Character Self-Evaluation</u>:

How would you describe your character? What do you need to improve upon, (hint we all can use improvement)? How can you take what you have learned here and begin the process of improvement?

Unit I LP 1. C. Personal Reflection:

Take the time to reflect on what you think will make you a good CNA. Write those qualities down here.

Ask yourself and answer the following question. "I want to be a good CNA because?"

Hint: Keep this answer where you can look at it as you go through the course. Are you achieving, learning, and applying the answers to your question?

***Unit I LP 1 D. Personal Reflection**: Utilizing the qualities that we just discussed write a paragraph of how you will utilize these qualities in your career as a Certified Nurse Assistant. Make a bullet point list.*

- *I will exhibit sensitivity to my residents by:* ____________________________
- *I will exhibit patience with my residents by:* ______________________________
- *I will be honest with my residents and co-workers by:* ______________________
- *I will present with a cheerful attitude at work by:* ____________________________
- *I will show my willingness at work by:* ______________________________________
- *I will demonstrate observation skills by:* ______________________________________
- *I will demonstrate reliability by:* ____
- *I will always exhibit a positive attitude by:* ________________________________

These should be a list you can keep where you can see it from time to time, your locker at work or some other place. Review it from time to time to see how you are doing. These become your goals for being the best CNA you can be!

Unit I LP 1 E. Review of Facility Hiring Practices:

Specifically look at what background checks employees must complete and what types of information in the background would prevent an offer of employment or result in termination. You will likely find this in the personnel manual or hiring manual. Ask a supervisor if you're unsure.

Unit I LP 1 F. Policy Review:

Ask to see the policies at the facility regarding these five key areas (infections, musculoskeletal injuries, stress, chemical exposure, and violence). If you are not sure what you're looking for ask a supervisor. If you have questions find a supervisor and ask them.

Unit I LP 2 Workbook Exercises

Unit I LP 1 G. Health and Habits

How would you rate your health and your habits of taking care of you? If you could pick one area that you could work on to improve, what would it be? Are you a smoker? Why do you smoke? Do you want to quit? Consider and write down ways you could move in that direction.

Unit I LP 2 Workbook Exercises

Unit I LP 2, A. Job Description:

Secure a copy of the CNA job description. You should have been provided a copy or at the very least reviewed it during orientation or through the hiring process.

1. Review it
2. Do you understand the duties and functions?
3. If not seek a supervisor for answers.

Unit I LP 2, B: Family Interview

Interview a family member regarding their feelings on the relationships they have with the resident and the staff of the facility. Reflect on ways you can incorporate what you learn from the interview into your practice.

Unit I LP 2 Workbook Exercises

Unit I LP 2 C. Quality of Life

Interview 3 residents about their life in the nursing home. Ask them to consider and answer the following questions.

1. What do you like about living in the nursing home? What do you not like?
2. Do you feel at home here? How could we make you feel more at home?
3. What are some things you miss about living in your home in the community? Could we fix that for you?

Unit I LP 2 D: Customer Service

1. Ask about how bathing preferences are incorporated into the care of the resident in the facility?
    a. Does the answer you receive meet your expectation of customer service? What could you do to assure that it does meet your expectation?
    b. Again, walk a mile in the other person's shoes, understand where they are coming from and then commit to making the journey a pleasure for them.
2. Observe a meal in the dining room. Consider our restaurant discussion in the lesson plan.
    a. What do you see that respects customer service?
    b. What do you see that needs some work?
    c. What could you do to get a better outcome if you were the one serving the residents at the meal?

Unit I LP 2 E. Patient Advocacy

1. Interview other team members and ask; "How do you advocate for the well-being of your patients/residents? "(interview at least one other CNA, and one each from Dietary, Activities and Social Services)
2. You are assigned a resident who a CNA tells you sexually assaulted his grandchildren, and the family could no longer manage his dementia (confusion) at home, so they admitted him to the nursing home. The family is angry at him and have not been to see him. He does not remember doing anything inappropriate and can't understand why he has been "left here to die."
   a. First, how are you feeling about taking care of him?
   b. Second, how are you going to advocate for him?
   c. What other team members need to be aware of how he is feeling?

Unit I LP 3. A: Listen to a report.

1. Did report stay on task or did staff talk about other things besides the residents?
2. What did you learn that you would need to incorporate into your duties if the residents were assigned to you?
3. Would you have the information you needed to confidently take care of the residents if they were assigned to you?
4. How long did report take?
5. Who participated?

Unit I LP 3 B. Personnel Policy Disciplinary Action or Grounds for Termination Review

Review in the Personnel manual the grounds for termination or disciplinary action. Talk to your supervisor if you are unsure what would be considered grounds for disciplinary action or have questions on what you have read.

Unit I LP 3 C: Review Dress Code and Observe Professionalism

1. Go to the personnel manual and review dress code and any other sections around what we have talked about here (code of ethics, behaviors, etc.)
2. Observe staff through nursing and other departments. Based on what you learned write down what you observed and the impressions you had about professionalism while observing.

Unit I LP 3. D: Applied Knowledge

A co-worker and a person you consider a friend is working on the hall with you today. She suggests that you do not do your showers today, even though they were assigned by the charge nurse. Instead, you help her do hers and she will help you do yours tomorrow. You agree if the charge nurse approves. She does not want to involve the charge nurse. She says she'll chart yours like they are done so you don't have to, and no one will be the wiser.

1. What qualities of a CNA is she asking you to ignore?
2. What actions is she suggesting that could result in disciplinary action?
3. What type of behavior do you need to use to make it clear that you cannot do as she asks?

Reflection/Answer

1. She is asking you to ignore reliability. Your charge nurse and residents are depending on you to provide the care they need as assigned not when it is convenient for staff. You may also be demonstrating, she certainly is, that you are not sensitive to the needs of a resident to feel clean and fresh when they cannot meet that need on their own.

2. Being negligent in the performance of duties, charting fraudulent documentation, insubordination or disobedience to a charge nurse and behavior that violates residents'' rights or affects care. These are all potential violations that could result in legal and/or disciplinary action.

3. Assertive Behavior- I cannot do what you ask, here is why and if you persist this is what I will have to do about it.

Becoming a Certified Nurse Assistant: A Person-Centered Approach

Unit I LP 2 Workbook Exercises

Applied Knowledge

A co-worker and a person you consider a friend is working on the hall with you today. She suggests that you do not do your showers today, even though they were assigned by the charge nurse. Instead, you help her do hers and she will help you do yours tomorrow. You agree if the charge nurse approves. She does not want to involve the charge nurse. She says she will chart yours like they are done so you don't have to, and no one will be the wiser.

1. What qualities of a CNA is she asking you to ignore?
2. What actions is she suggesting that could result in disciplinary action?
3. What type of behavior do you need to use to make it clear that you cannot do as she asks?

Reflection/Answer

1. She is asking you to ignore reliability. Your charge nurse and residents are depending on you to provide the care they need as assigned not when it is convenient for staff. You may also be demonstrating, she certainly is, that you are not sensitive to the needs of a resident to feel clean and fresh when they cannot meet that need on their own.

2. Being negligent in the performance of duties, charting fraudulent documentation, insubordination or disobedience to a charge nurse and behavior that violates residents'' rights or affects care. These are all potential violations that could result in legal and/or disciplinary action.

3. Assertive Behavior- I cannot do what you ask, here is why and if you persist this is what I will have to do about it.

Becoming a Certified Nurse Assistant: A Person-Centered Approach

Unit II Workbook Exercises

Unit II LP 1 A: Ethical Decision Making using the PLUS Model

In the example of the CNA not taking the vital signs described in Lesson Plan 1. Let's look at the plus model and work through this using it as a tool to help us make the right decision.

A team member (another CNA) does not do her vital signs but hands a list of vital signs to the charge nurse, claiming that she did them. You know she did not and in fact when you question her, she tells you; "I didn't have time. They are not important anyway everyone is fine. They are just routine. Please do not say anything. I really need this job!"

The PLUS Model:

- P = Policies and Procedures (Does this decision align with company policies? When in doubt ask.)
- L = Legal (Does this decision violate any laws or regulations? When in doubt ask.)
- U = Universal (Is this decision in line with core values of the facility? When in doubt ask.)
- S = Self (Does it meet my standards of fairness and honesty? When in doubt reflect.)

1. What does the policy and procedure manual say about vital signs?
2. What does it say about failure to perform an assigned duty?
3. Does the decision that the CNA made violate any laws or regulations? (Remember when in doubt ask.)
4. Does the decision lineup with facility values? (Remember when in doubt ask.
5. Does the decision meet your standard of fairness and honesty?

Now work through the Ethical Decision-Making Process

1. Step One: Define the Problem (how did it violate the PLUS acronyms)
2. Step Two: Seek Out Resources (what resources did you use)
3. Step Three: Brainstorm a List of Potential Solutions (what are your options)
4. Step Four: Evaluate Those Alternatives (what are the potential impacts of the decisions your considering)
5. Step Five: Make Your Decision, and Implement It (what is your decision)
6. Step Six: Evaluate Your Decision (why is your decision the best solution)

Reflection:

Problem Defined: This CNA violated policy and procedure, code of practice, lied, placed resident's in harm's way and was illegal (neglect). Her actions should violate the facility values and your own.

The resources used to come to this conclusion would include facility policy and procedure, employee handbook on conduct, nursing code of ethics, and regulatory guidance (you likely at th is stage would need help finding how this violates regulation).

Potential Solutions and their evaluation include

1) *Not doing anything and risking that she will not do it again or that someone (a resident) may get hurt in the process*

2) *Reporting your firsthand knowledge to the charge nurse or supervisor and allowing them to put the steps into motion for disciplinary action and assuring the residents are indeed okay.*

3) *Talking to the CNA yourself about how this violates ethical practice, offering to help her get the vital signs and then letting her come up with some story about how the first set was wrong.) However, do you have any faith that she will not do something similar again? What risk does that pose to residents?*

Make and evaluate your decision

The best solution here is number 2 above. You know she lied about critical information that could place residents at risk. Regardless that you like her the behavior and actions were unethical, illegal, and potentially harmful to the residents. Your honesty and integrity are now on the line just because of your awareness of the facts.

Unit II, LP 3 B. Abuse and Neglect Policy and Procedure

Ask to review the facility Policy and Procedure for Abuse and Neglect and then answer these questions:

1. What are my responsibilities as a CNA in monitoring for and reporting abuse?
2. What actions might be considered abuse by a CNA?
3. What physical and behavior signs of abuse should I monitor for?
4. What do I do if I suspect a resident is being abused or neglected?
5. What do I do if I see a resident being abused or neglected?
6. Who do I contact if I suspect or witness abuse or neglect?

Unit II, LP 4 A. Review of Statement of Deficiencies

All long-term care facilities are required to post their last statement of deficiencies in a place where residents and families or visitors can review them. Ask the facility where their copy of the last survey results is (Statement of Deficiencies) review them now. If you have any questions, ask the supervisor.

Unit II, LP 4 B. DON Interview

Ask the Director of Nurses for some time to interview him/her about the survey process.

1. What is their expectation of you when surveyors are in the facility?
2. How do they want you to answer questions if the surveyor asks?
3. If you have a concern about something a surveyor asked you who do they want you to talk to about it?

Unit II LP 5 A Dignity Violations Feelings and Reflections

Recall a situation in which you felt that your personal dignity was violated.

1. Describe here what happened and how you felt when the event occurred.
2. How do you feel about it now?
3. Did you have any strong or overpowering emotions (shame, anger/rage, powerlessness, frustration, sadness, disgust, a feeling of uncleanliness or hopelessness?

Remember you probably lived in a dignity-supportive environment when you experienced this significant and memorable life event. Hopefully, you had support and efforts were made to assure it did not happen again.

1. How then might the quality and duration of impact differ for people who live in an environment characterized by severe, sustained, institutionalized and repetitive violations?
2. Have you seen examples of potentially repetitive dignity violations in the facility?
3. What were they?
4. How might the resident be feeling about these?

Unit III LP 2. A Care Plan Review

Ask to review a resident's care plan and any communication tools the facility may use for the CNA, such as an abbreviated version.

1. What did you learn about the resident?
2. What approaches were items you would need to incorporate into your daily approach to care of the individual?
3. What areas of resident condition would you want to observe and report changes in that could impact this care plan?

Unit III LP 2 B. CNA Charting Review

Look at the ADL sheets for 5 residents. Record what you see as errors from what we've learned here.

Unit II, LP 5 B. Self-Reflection-Your Habits, Preferences and Routines

1. Describe what you do when you get up in the morning to prepare for your day? Which of those things, as you reflect, have become habits and routines? Which are rituals? Why are they important to your quality of life? What happens to your quality of life if you are no longer able to do them?
2. Describe what you do to relax and unwind in the evening and then your bedtime routine? Which of those things, as you reflect, have become habits and routines? Which are rituals? Why are they important to your quality of life? What happens to your quality of life if you are no longer able to do them?

Unit II LP 5 C. Self-Reflection: Designing Your Own Person-Centered Care

You will be admitted as a resident tomorrow. You don't know yet whether it will be a short stay or longer, maybe even permeant.

1. Consider your own history, preferences, routines, and habits around the **activities of daily living** that we all perform for ourselves daily. Someone will have to help you with them now. What do you want your caregiver to know about so that your care is person-centered?
    a. Bathing Routines
    b. Sleeping Routines
    c. Grooming Routines
    d. Dining and Food Routines
    e. Exercise or physical activity routines
    f. How you get around (transfer yourself, etc.)
    g. Toileting (stress incontinence-how do you manage it?)
2. Consider your relationships with people (family, friends, community) and what your social activities have been, what you do for fun and really enjoy. What do you want your caregiver to know about so that your care is person-centered?
    a. Games and hobbies
    b. Relationships that are important (family, friends, clubs or groups you are a member of)

Becoming a Certified Nurse Assistant: A Person-Centered Approach

Unit III LP 1 A. Terms and Abbreviations Matching Exercise

Name: Meagan A.

Abbreviations

Write the letter of the correct match next to each problem.

Created on TheTeachersCorner.net Match-up Maker

1. f	A	a.	Activity of Daily Living
2. j	a.c.	b.	Bowel Movement
3. r	Abd	c.	amount
4. p	Ad Lib	d.	Bedside Commode
5. a	ADL	e.	Bathroom privledges
6. n	adm	f.	Before
7. s	AM	g.	With
8. o	amb.	h.	Apical
9. c	amt.	i.	capsule
10. h	AP	j.	Before Meals
11. q	ASAP	k.	Bedrest
12. l	b,i,d	l.	twice per day
13. b	BM	m.	Blood Pressure
14. m	B/P or BP	n.	Admission
15. k	BR	o.	Ambulate
16. e	BRP	p.	At will, As desired, at liberty
17. d	BSC	q.	As soon as possible
18. g	c (with line over)	r.	Abdomen
19. t	cath	s.	Morning
20. i	cap	t.	catheter

Name:__________________

Abbreviations

Write the letter of the correct match next to each problem.

	Answer	Abbreviation		Meaning
1.	f	A	a.	Activity of Daily Living
2.	j	a.c.	b.	Bowel Movement
3.	r	Abd	c.	amount
4.	p	Ad Lib	d.	Bedside Commode
5.	a	ADL	e.	Bathroom privledges
6.	n	adm	f.	Before
7.	s	AM	g.	With
8.	o	amb.	h.	Apical
9.	c	amt.	i.	capsule
10.	h	AP	j.	Before Meals
11.	q	ASAP	k.	Bedrest
12.	l	b,i,d	l.	twice per day
13.	b	BM	m.	Blood Pressure
14.	m	B/P or BP	n.	Admission
15.	k	BR	o.	Ambulate
16.	e	BRP	p.	At will, As desired, at liberty
17.	d	BSC	q.	As soon as possible
18.	g	c (with line over)	r.	Abdomen
19.	t	cath	s.	Morning
20.	i	cap	t.	catheter

Becoming a Certified Nurse Assistant: A Person-Centered Approach

Matching Abbreviations to Meaning

Name:________________

Abbreviations 2

Write the letter of the correct match next to each problem.

1. ______	cc	a. Carbon Dioxide
2. ______	c/o	b. electrocardiogram
3. ______	CO2	c. Cardiopulmonary resuscitation
4. ______	CPR	d. complains of
5. ______	CVA	e. Estimted Blood Loss
6. ______	CXR	f. fracture
7. ______	d/c	g. Director of Nurses
8. ______	DON	h. cubic centimeter
9. ______	Drsg or dsg	i. Foot
10. ______	dx	j. discontinue or discharge
11. ______	ECG or EKG	k. cerebrovascular accident: stroke
12. ______	EBL	l. Diagnosis
13. ______	ER	m. Force fluids
14. ______	F	n. Fahrenheit
15. ______	FF	o. Emergency Room
16. ______	ft.	p. dressing
17. ______	fb	q. Chest X-ray
18. ______	fx	r. drop-liquid measurement
19. ______	gttt	s. hour
20. ______	h or hr	t. foreign body

Name:__________________

Abbreviations 2

Write the letter of the correct match next to each problem.

#	Answer	Abbreviation		Meaning
1.	h	cc	a.	Carbon Dioxide
2.	d	c/o	b.	electrocardiogram
3.	a	CO2	c.	Cardiopulmonary resuscitation
4.	c	CPR	d.	complains of
5.	k	CVA	e.	Estimted Blood Loss
6.	q	CXR	f.	fracture
7.	j	d/c	g.	Director of Nurses
8.	g	DON	h.	cubic centimeter
9.	p	Drsg or dsg	i.	Foot
10.	l	dx	j.	discontinue or discharge
11.	b	ECG or EKG	k.	cerebrovascular accident: stroke
12.	e	EBL	l.	Diagnosis
13.	o	ER	m.	Force fluids
14.	n	F	n.	Fahrenheit
15.	m	FF	o.	Emergency Room
16.	i	ft.	p.	dressing
17.	t	fb	q.	Chest X-ray
18.	f	fx	r.	drop-liquid measurement
19.	r	gttt	s.	hour
20.	s	h or hr	t.	foreign body

Becoming a Certified Nurse Assistant: A Person-Centered Approach

Name: ____________________

Write the letter of the correct match next to each problem.

1.	________	H2O	a. intramuscular
2.	________	HA	b. 1
3.	________	HOH	c. 4
4.	________	H & P	d. height
5.	________	HR	e. intravenous
6.	________	hs	f. Hard of hearing
7.	________	ht	g. insulin dependent diabetes mellitus
8.	________	i	h. medical doctor
9.	________	ii	i. water
10.	________	iii	j. 2
11.	________	iv	k. 3
12.	________	v	l. Headache
13.	________	I & O	m. Intradisciplinary care plan
14.	________	ICP	n. kilogram (2.2 kg=1 lb.)
15.	________	IDDM	o. hour of sleep (bedtime)
16.	________	IV	p. intake and output
17.	________	IM	q. history and physical
18.	________	kg	r. heart rate
19.	________	l or lt	s. 5
20.	________	MD	t. left

Becoming a Certified Nurse Assistant: A Person-Centered Approach

Name:__________________

Write the letter of the correct match next to each problem.

#	Answer	Term	Match
1.	i	H2O	a. intramuscular
2.	l	HA	b. 1
3.	f	HOH	c. 4
4.	q	H & P	d. height
5.	r	HR	e. intravenous
6.	o	hs	f. Hard of hearing
7.	d	ht	g. insulin dependent diabetes mellitus
8.	b	i	h. medical doctor
9.	j	ii	i. water
10.	k	iii	j. 2
11.	c	iv	k. 3
12.	s	v	l. Headache
13.	p	I & O	m. Intradisciplinary care plan
14.	m	ICP	n. kilogram (2.2 kg=1 lb.)
15.	g	IDDM	o. hour of sleep (bedtime)
16.	e	IV	p. intake and output
17.	a	IM	q. history and physical
18.	n	kg	r. heart rate
19.	t	l or lt	s. 5
20.	h	MD	t. left

Becoming a Certified Nurse Assistant: A Person-Centered Approach

Name:__________________

Write the letter of the correct match next to each problem.

1. ________	NPO	a. postoperative (after surgery)
2. ________	noc	b. Physical Therapy
3. ________	O2	c. Per rectum
4. ________	OD	d. Afternoon or evening
5. ________	OS	e. after meals
6. ________	OU	f. both eyes
7. ________	OOB	g. Out of bed
8. ________	OT	h. after
9. ________	p	i. oxygen
10. ________	PM	j. left eye
11. ________	po	k. every day
12. ________	PR	l. occupational therapy
13. ________	post-op	m. night
14. ________	pre-op	n. patient
15. ________	pt	o. preoperative (before surgery)
16. ________	prn	p. every
17. ________	pc	q. nothing by mouth
18. ________	PT	r. right eye
19. ________	q	s. as needed
20. ________	qd	t. by mouth

Becoming a Certified Nurse Assistant: A Person-Centered Approach

Name:________________

Write the letter of the correct match next to each problem.

#	Answer	Term		Definition
1.	q	NPO	a.	postoperative (after surgery)
2.	m	noc	b.	Physical Therapy
3.	i	O2	c.	Per rectum
4.	r	OD	d.	Afternoon or evening
5.	j	OS	e.	after meals
6.	f	OU	f.	both eyes
7.	g	OOB	g.	Out of bed
8.	l	OT	h.	after
9.	h	p	i.	oxygen
10.	d	PM	j.	left eye
11.	t	po	k.	every day
12.	c	PR	l.	occupational therapy
13.	a	post-op	m.	night
14.	o	pre-op	n.	patient
15.	n	pt	o.	preoperative (before surgery)
16.	s	prn	p.	every
17.	e	pc	q.	nothing by mouth
18.	b	PT	r.	right eye
19.	p	q	s.	as needed
20.	k	qd	t.	by mouth

Becoming a Certified Nurse Assistant: A Person-Centered Approach

Name:________________

Write the letter of the correct match next to each problem.

1.	______	qh	a.	Range of Motion
2.	______	qhs	b.	subcutaneous
3.	______	qid	c.	every 2 hours, every 3 hours, every 4 hours, etc.
4.	______	qod	d.	every hour
5.	______	q2h, q3h, q4h, etc.	e.	symptoms
6.	______	R or rt	f.	immediately
7.	______	RCP	g.	four times a day
8.	______	res	h.	without
9.	______	ROM	i.	short of breath
10.	______	RX	j.	every hour of sleep
11.	______	sc/sq	k.	right
12.	______	s	l.	resident
13.	______	sx	m.	Resident care plan
14.	______	s/s	n.	specimen
15.	______	stat	o.	every other day
16.	______	SOB	p.	three times a day
17.	______	spec	q.	prescription, treatment
18.	______	tab	r.	tablet
19.	______	tid	s.	signs and symptoms
20.	______	TPR	t.	temperature, pulse, respiration

Becoming a Certified Nurse Assistant: A Person-Centered Approach

Name:________________

Write the letter of the correct match next to each problem.

#	Answer	Term		Definition
1.	d	qh	a.	Range of Motion
2.	j	qhs	b.	subcutaneous
3.	g	qid	c.	every 2 hours, every 3 hours, every 4 hours, etc.
4.	o	qod	d.	every hour
5.	c	q2h, q3h, q4h, etc.	e.	symptoms
6.	k	R or rt	f.	immediately
7.	m	RCP	g.	four times a day
8.	l	res	h.	without
9.	a	ROM	i.	short of breath
10.	q	RX	j.	every hour of sleep
11.	b	sc/sq	k.	right
12.	h	s	l.	resident
13.	e	sx	m.	Resident care plan
14.	s	s/s	n.	specimen
15.	f	stat	o.	every other day
16.	i	SOB	p.	three times a day
17.	n	spec	q.	prescription, treatment
18.	r	tab	r.	tablet
19.	p	tid	s.	signs and symptoms
20.	t	TPR	t.	temperature, pulse, respiration

Workbook Exercise

Unit III LP 4 A. Temperature Skills

Gather supplies and use the competency sheet to check the temperature of at least 4 co-workers. Have them check to see if you have it right. When you are ready find your clinical supervisor or RN Instructor and tell him/her you are ready to take an oral temperature using a glass thermometer. Repeat this exercise for rectal (ask which residents may need a rectal temp, -your co-workers are not likely to volunteer for this one), axillary, tympanic and temporal forehead temperature. Once a competency sheet is completed, signed off indicating you have the skill to do the procedure competently, ask the instructor/clinical supervisor if you are to keep them or they are retained by them until you have them all completed. There completion will have to be documented, including the date and who reviewed it, for final submission to the state for certification (in most states).

Unit III LP 4 B. Pulse Skills

Gather supplies and use the competency sheet to check the pulses of at least 4 co-workers. Have them check to see if you have it right. Do this for radial and apical pulse. Once a competency sheet is completed, signed off indicating you have the skill to do the procedure competently, ask the instructor/clinical supervisor if you are to keep them or they are retained by them until you have them all completed. There completion will have to be documented, including the date and who reviewed it, for final submission to the state for certification (in most states).

Unit III LP 4 C. Respiratory Skills

Gather supplies and use the competency sheet to check the respirations of at least 4 co-workers. Have them check to see if you have it right. Once a competency sheet is completed, signed off indicating you have the skill to do the procedure competently, ask the instructor/clinical supervisor if you are to keep them or they are retained by them until you have them all completed. There completion will have to be documented, including the date and who reviewed it, for final submission to the state for certification (in most states).

Unit III LP 4 D. Blood Pressure Skills

Gather supplies and use the competency sheet to check the blood pressure of at least 4 co-workers. Have them check to see if you have it right. Once a competency sheet is completed, signed off indicating you have the skill to do the procedure competently, ask the instructor/clinical supervisor if you are to keep them or they are retained by them until you have them all completed. There completion will have to be documented, including the date and who reviewed it, for final submission to the state for certification (in most states).

Unit III LP 4 E. Pulse Oximetry Skills

Gather supplies and use the competency sheet to check the pulse oximetry of at least 4 co-workers. Have them check to see if you have it right. Once a competency sheet is completed, signed off indicating you have the skill to do the procedure competently, ask the instructor/clinical supervisor if you are to keep them or they are retained by them until you have them all completed. There completion will have to be documented, including the date and who reviewed it, for final submission to the state for certification (in most states).

Unit III LP 4 F. Height and Weight Skills

Gather supplies and use the competency sheet to check the height and weight of at least 4 co-workers. Have them check to see if you have it right. Once a competency sheet is completed, signed off indicating you have the skill to do the procedure competently, ask the instructor/clinical supervisor if you are to keep them or they are retained by them until you have them all completed. There completion will have to be documented, including the date and who reviewed it, for final submission to the state for certification (in most states).

Becoming a Certified Nurse Assistant: A Person-Centered Approach

Name:___________________

Mental Health

Complete the crossword puzzle below

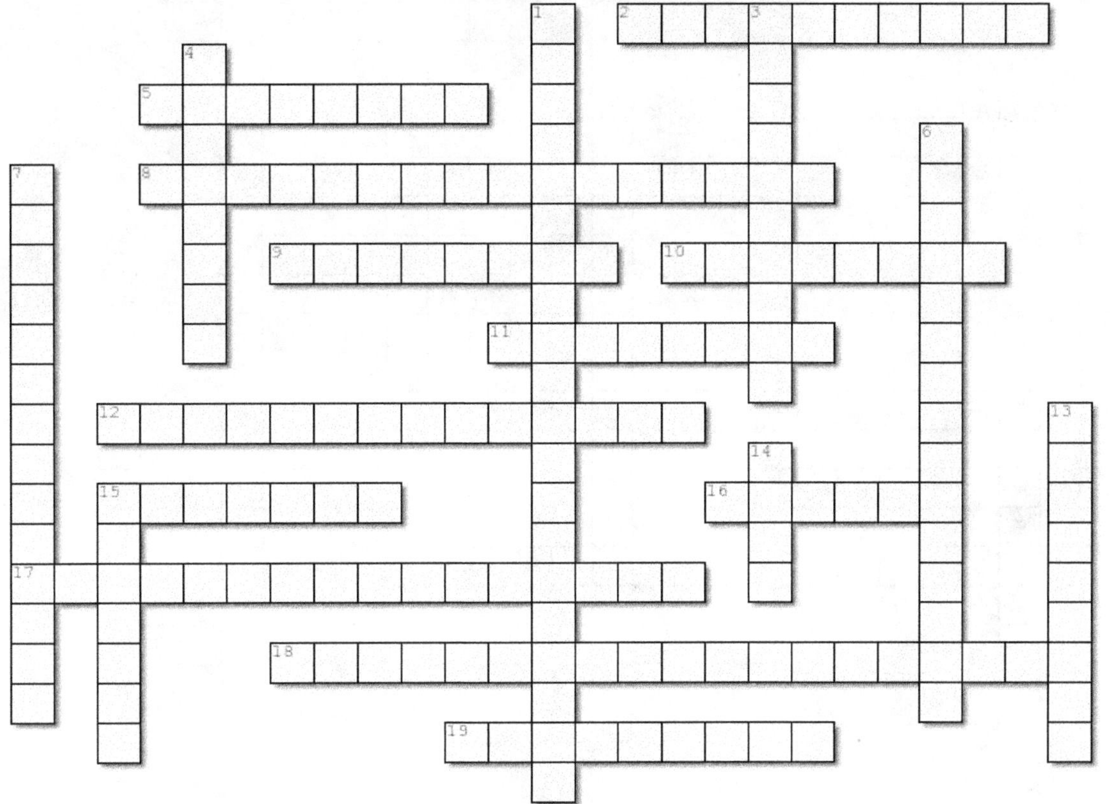

Created using the Crossword Maker on TheTeachersCorner.net

Across

2. phenomenon when confusion becomes worse in the evening
5. severe impairment of cognitive functions such as thinking, memory, and personally; comes on slowly and worsens over time
8. brain disorders that cause changes in a person's mood, energy and ability to function
9. suspiciousness inappropriate to reality; individual feels that everyone is picking on him/her or out to get him/her
10. habitual sleeplessness; inability to sleep
11. false thought that a person believes to be real
12. sensory perceptions that seem real to the person experiencing them but are not perceived by others
15. apprehensive uneasiness or nervousness usually over an impending or anticipated event.
16. a state of mental or emotional strain or tension resulting from adverse or very demanding circumstances
17. Managing pain, behaviors or other symptoms without medication
18. a progress impairment of memory, reasoning, and judgement that is related to cellular changes within the brain and that leads
19. aimless walking, which may result in a resident becoming lost

Down

1. measurable decline in memory and thinking skills
3. a mood disorder that causes a persistent feeling of sadness and loss of interest
4. memory and thinking impairment that comes on suddenly and is caused by illness or toxic reactions in the body, usually revers
6. a mental disorder defined by abnormal eating habits that negatively affect a person's physical or mental health.
7. behavioral or mental pattern that causes significant distress or impairment of personal functioning
13. the patient leaving a facility without notice or staff awareness
14. Involves the development of symptoms following exposure to one or more traumatic, life-threatening events
15. loss of the ability to recognize familiar objects

Becoming a Certified Nurse Assistant: A Person-Centered Approach

Name:___________________

Mental Health

Complete the crossword puzzle below

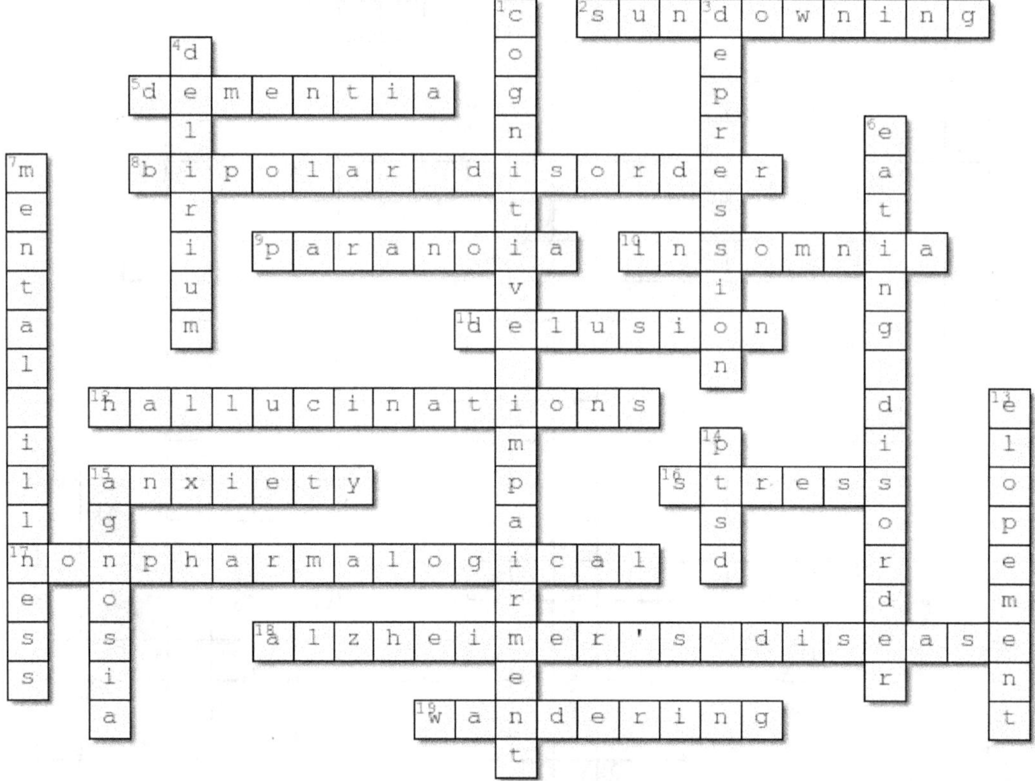

Created using the Crossword Maker on TheTeachersCorner.net

Across

2. phenomenon when confusion becomes worse in the evening (**sundowning**)
5. severe impairment of cognitive functions such as thinking, memory, and personally; comes on slowly and worsens over time (**dementia**)
8. brain disorders that cause changes in a person's mood, energy and ability to function (**bipolar disorder**)
9. suspiciousness inappropriate to reality; individual feels that everyone is picking on him/her or out to get him/her (**paranoia**)
10. habitual sleeplessness; inability to sleep (**insomnia**)
11. false thought that a person believes to be real (**delusion**)
12. sensory perceptions that seem real to the person experiencing them but are not perceived by others (**hallucinations**)
15. apprehensive uneasiness or nervousness usually over an impending or anticipated event. (**anxiety**)
16. a state of mental or emotional strain or tension resulting from adverse or very demanding circumstances (**stress**)
17. Managing pain, behaviors or other symptoms without medication (**nonpharmalogical**)
18. a progress impairment of memory, reasoning, and judgement that is related to cellular changes within the brain and that leads (**alzheimer's disease**)
19. aimless walking, which may result in a resident becoming lost (**wandering**)

Down

1. measurable decline in memory and thinking skills (**cognitive impairment**)
3. a mood disorder that causes a persistent feeling of sadness and loss of interest (**depression**)
4. memory and thinking impairment that comes on suddenly and is caused by illness or toxic reactions in the body, usually revers (**delirium**)
6. a mental disorder defined by abnormal eating habits that negatively affect a person's physical or mental health. (**eating disorder**)
7. behavioral or mental pattern that causes significant distress or impairment of personal functioning (**mental illness**)
13. the patient leaving a facility without notice or staff awareness (**elopement**)
14. Involves the development of symptoms following exposure to one or more traumatic, life-threatening events (**ptsd**)
15. loss of the ability to recognize familiar objects (**agnosia**)

Name:________________

Observations of Mental Health

D W T J O W O Q N V R P S Q H G G C Z U
Z I Z N G U T H M B U U W Y T J K A A N
U S Z O S H R C D A G X A C X C E J B X
Q H Y I H T I G G N I N W O D N U S N M
Y F G I T O W I Z Q B E H A V I O R J G
L T A Q N D A C D S T F J U C T J L L C
Z F U D E L U S I O N Z A G W Z U V B K
L T E D M B D Z T L L M A O B L N G I H
T P S R E G G I R T L H B J J K H F O T
D Y R Q P J F C O M M U N I C A T I O N
S U O S O Q T L U U G A S T J A T P Z V
D D X V L V B X L J B H U Y W D T O R E
L R R G E V I T C E T O R P P O A D T I
T B A J G R D K E J O W A E K J U U V U
G J W T B D S R V E V I C C V A C C D C
T G R K E X N I G N I R E D N A W C V O
M T H D M X V S G B I D O R Z U L A O D
S S U Y L A Q V D H L D D E L I R I U M
S Z W W N U H E S M T D X R O G T U F W
B O A H L E N N N C I N O R H C O P K C

ACUTE	BEHAVIOR	CHRONIC
COMMUNICATION	DELIRIUM	DELUSION
ELOPEMENT	OVERSIGHT	PROTECTIVE
SUNDOWNING	TRIGGERS	WANDERING

Becoming a Certified Nurse Assistant: A Person-Centered Approach

Name:________________

Created with TheTeachersCorner.net Word Search Maker

Observations of Mental Health

D W T J O W O Q N V R P S Q H G G C Z U

Z I Z N G U T H M B U U W Y T J K A A N

U S Z O S H R C D A G X A C X C E J B X

Q H Y I H T I G G N I N W O D N U S N M

Y F G I T O W I Z Q B E H A V I O R J G

L T A Q N D A C D S T F J U C T J L L C

Z F U D E L U S I O N Z A G W Z U V B K

L T E D M B D Z T L L M A O B L N G I H

T P S R E G G I R T L H B J J K H F O T

D Y R Q P J F C O M M U N I C A T I O N

S U O S O Q T L U U G A S T J A T P Z V

D D X V L V B X L J B H U Y W D T O R E

L R R G E V I T C E T O R P P O A D T I

T B A J G R D K E J O W A E K J U U V U

G J W T B D S R V E V I C C V A C C D C

T G R K E X N I G N I R E D N A W C V O

M T H D M X V S G B I D O R Z U L A O D

S S U Y L A Q V D H L D D E L I R I U M

S Z W W N U H E S M T D X R O G T U F W

B O A H L E N N N C I N O R H C O P K C

ACUTE	BEHAVIOR	CHRONIC
COMMUNICATION	DELIRIUM	DELUSION
ELOPEMENT	OVERSIGHT	PROTECTIVE
SUNDOWNING	TRIGGERS	WANDERING

Unit V Human Anatomy & Physiology-The Impact of Aging

Workbook Exercise LP I

Ask the charge nurse or DON about the facility policy on pressure ulcer prevention. Ask to see it, read it and ask any questions you don't understand. Then ask for permission to do rounds with the wound nurse to see any pressure ulcers or wounds and how they are treated. Ask questions such as:

1. How did this happen?
2. What could prevent it?

Unit VI LP 1 Worksheet Exercise 1

Review 10 incident reports and answer the following:

1. What were most of the incidents about (falls, altercations, wandering, etc.)?
2. Did the report give you enough information to determine what might have caused the incident?
3. Did any incident involve equipment malfunction or misuse? If so, what did you learn from reviewing it?
4. Who completed the report? Were there additional statements included or referenced from other staff such as a CNA?

Unit VI LP 1 Worksheet Exercise 2

Review the facility policy and procedure on fire safety and the CNA's role. Are you comfortable you know what to do in a fire emergency?

Unit VI LP 2 Worksheet Exercise 1

Complete the RACE Fill in the blank in the workbook.

Name:__________________

RACE- Complete the Senteance

Use the words in the list below to complete the sentence

Created on TheTeachersCorner.net Fill-in-the-Blank Maker

CLEAR	ACTIVATE
REMOVE	EXTINGUISH

1. Immediately __________ the resident from danger
2. Once the resident is safe, __________ the alarm
3. Once the alarm is sounded __________ the area and follow the evacuation plan as practiced. Close doors to resident rooms and ensure that smoke doors are closed.
4. If safe, __________ the fire with the approved extinguisher

Name:__________________

RACE- Complete the Senteance

Use the words in the list below to complete the sentence

Created on TheTeachersCorner.net Fill-in-the-Blank Maker

CLEAR	ACTIVATE
REMOVE	EXTINGUISH

1. Immediately REMOVE the resident from danger
2. Once the resident is safe, ACTIVATE the alarm
3. Once the alarm is sounded CLEAR the area and follow the evacuation plan as practiced. Close doors to resident rooms and ensure that smoke doors are closed.
4. If safe, EXTINGUISH the fire with the approved extinguisher

Unit VI Lesson Plan 3. Ergonomic Rules of Safety Word Scramble

Name:________________

Ergonomics

Please unscramble the words below

1. siiAvesst evceDi ____________________
2. Byod caeinhscM ____________________
3. corosEmign ____________________
4. atiG letB ____________________
5. cenaMhalic Lfit ____________________
6. letluMelosacuks yrnluj ____________________
7. Tsrnerfa oaBdr ____________________

Name:________________

Ergonomics

Please unscramble the words below

1. siiAvesst evceDi — Assistive Device
2. Byod caeinhscM — Body Mechanics
3. corosEmign — Ergonomics
4. atiG letB — Gait Belt
5. cenaMhalic Lfit — Mechanical Lift
6. letluMelosacuks yrnluj — Musculoskeletal Injury
7. Tsrnerfa oaBdr — Transfer Board

LP VII LP Workbook Exercise I

Workbook Exercise

Review the facility policy and procedure(s) on infection control. Locate the items that we have talked about within this lesson plan and that are discussed in the policy and procedure such as:

1. Gloves
2. Hand Sanitizers
3. Biohazard Sharps Containers
4. Gowns, Masks, Face, and Eye Protection

LP VII LP Workbook Exercise II

Observe 5 handwashing or gloving or both procedures by staff. Use your competency sheets and check off their skills. How did they do? What did they do well? What did they do wrong?

Becoming a Certified Nurse Assistant: A Person-Centered Approach

LP VII LP Workbook Exercise

Name:________________

Write the letter of the correct match next to each problem.

Created on TheTeachersCorner.net Match-up Maker

1. ________	Communicable disease	a. microbes that cause disease
2. ________	Community-acquired i	b. organism that lives in or on another organism
3. ________	Culture & Sensitivit	c. sudden increase in cases of a disease within a certain geographic area or within a facility, school, community, etc.
4. ________	Healthcare-associate	d. sample of fluid or tissue taken for examination and/or testing
5. ________	Multi-drug resistant	e. infections that are present or incubating at the time of admission and which generally develop within 72 hours of admission.
6. ________	Outbreak	f. an infection that residents acquire, that is associated with a medical or surgical intervention (e.g., podiatry, wound care d
7. ________	Parasite:	g. microbes—bacteria, fungi, viruses, or parasites—that have evolved immunity to one or more of the drugs used to kill them.
8. ________	Pathogens	h. an infection transmissible (e.g., from person-to-person) by direct contact with an affected individual or the individual's bo
9. ________	Resistant organisms	i. a test to find germs (such as bacteria or a fungus) that can cause an infection. A sensitivity test checks to see what kind o
10. ________	Specimen	j.): microorganisms, predominantly bacteria, that are resistant to one or more antimicrobial agents, and are usually resistant
11. ________	Urinalysis	k. physical, chemical and microscopic examination of a urine sample
12. ________	Sputum	l. mixture of saliva and mucus coughed up from the respiratory tract, typically as a result of infection or other disease and of

Becoming a Certified Nurse Assistant: A Person-Centered Approach

Name:________________

Write the letter of the correct match next to each problem.

Created on TheTeachersCorner.net Match-up Maker

#	Answer	Term	Definition
1.	h	Communicable disease	a. microbes that cause disease
2.	e	Community-acquired i	b. organism that lives in or on another organism
3.	i	Culture & Sensitivit	c. sudden increase in cases of a disease within a certain geographic area or within a facility, school, community, etc.
4.	f	Healthcare-associate	d. sample of fluid or tissue taken for examination and/or testing
5.	j	Multi-drug resistant	e. infections that are present or incubating at the time of admission and which generally develop within 72 hours of admission.
6.	c	Outbreak	f. an infection that residents acquire, that is associated with a medical or surgical intervention (e.g., podiatry, wound care d
7.	b	Parasite:	g. microbes—bacteria, fungi, viruses, or parasites—that have evolved immunity to one or more of the drugs used to kill them.
8.	a	Pathogens	h. an infection transmissible (e.g., from person-to-person) by direct contact with an affected individual or the individual's bo
9.	g	Resistant organisms	i. a test to find germs (such as bacteria or a fungus) that can cause an infection. A sensitivity test checks to see what kind o
10.	d	Specimen	j.): microorganisms, predominantly bacteria, that are resistant to one or more antimicrobial agents, and are usually resistant
11.	k	Urinalysis	k. physical, chemical and microscopic examination of a urine sample
12.	l	Sputum	l. mixture of saliva and mucus coughed up from the respiratory tract, typically as a result of infection or other disease and of

Unit VIII LP 1 Workbook Exercise

Observe one meal without feeding in the dining room. Watch the interaction between residents, between resident and staff and observe the atmosphere.

1. Would you consider the service you observed as worthy of being tippable if we could accept tips? Yes or No, if not why?
2. Did staff talk to residents or each other mostly?
3. Did you observe good infection control practices?
4. Were residents being offered and encouraged to drink?
5. Did staff who were feeding residents:
    a. offer sips of fluids before starting?
    b. Identify foods as they were offered?
    c. Try to interact with the resident beyond the action of feeding someone?
    d. Keep the resident well-groomed during the process?
6. What did you notice about the overall atmosphere that you thought was pleasant?
7. What did you notice about the overall atmosphere that you did not find pleasant?

Unit IX Workbook Exercises

Failure to perform perineal care correctly is one of the leading causes of Urinary Tract Infections in long term care and one of the leading deficiencies cited by survey teams in the nation. Usually it involves failure to wash hands or glove correctly or incorrect technique in cleansing the perineum (always front to back or cleanest to dirtiest). Review the competency sheet for perineal care with a catheter associated with the lesson plans in Unit IX. Perineal care without a catheter is the same except for the cleansing and care of the catheter tubing. Practice on 5 residents with an experienced CNA and when you have it down as the clinical supervisor to sign off on your being competent and then remember to always follow the procedure.

Becoming a Certified Nurse Assistant: A Person-Centered Approach

Unit XI Worksheet Exercise

Name: ____________

Restorative Nursing Word Search

J X V O C G V V F W V F N Q H M K Q I P
E N O I S N E T X E N O I T C U D B A W
M I F B D G U R Q F I R F K L N I C G U
E Q B X S Z N U Z T M P Q F K O V U H H
D T V G X D I U A P C U K W M I G G L K
J T L H N S R N F E P G Q W X S T Z A I
B E U A H P I A V J B P I B H N D D T Z
H Z G N P P Z O F E C A J X U E F N E H
B B F I U V U H F N R L Q S N T R O R R
E X R S G R A M Q A E S Y B G X O I A L
V L R N L D P R O N A T I O N E T X L P
E P Z O N A A J C W D C G O P R A E N G
R B Q I V O Q C E G Y B A D N E T L J V
S B I T L F H Z Y X V Z W M F P I F W Z
I M I C C H X A Z Z J I Z O W Y O I X W
O L I U W R Q I H J U O X I A H N M R T
N C P D J D E J F Y W M O F X B S Y A C
I R C D N N F R D X X N A O N Q P X Y T
N J E A E D O X T I Q A J S T F I A R F
H E O M I R Y H K X Z W B U T Z M E P M

ABDUCTION	ADDUCTION	EVERSION
EXTENSION	FLEXION	HYPEREXTENSION
INVERSION	LATERAL	PRONATION
ROTATION	SUPINATION	

Unit XII Workbook Exercises

There are a number of religions and cultural differences in how the end of life care process is observed. The internet is a great place to learn more. Search for how a resident who is Jewish, Muslim, Hindu, etc. might have different needs than someone who is Christian in this time of their life. While completing the search write down things you might have to consider in your practice as you care for them at this time in their lives.

Becoming a Certified Nurse Assistant: A Person-Centered Approach

Final Mock Written Exam

1. The process of checking a person into a health care facility is which of the following?
   A. Transfer
   B. Discharge
   C. Admission
   D. Adjustment Difficulty
2. Refers to the development of emotional and/or behavioral symptoms in response to an identifiable stressor(s) that has not been the resident's typical response to stressors in the past or an inability to adjust to stressors as evidenced by chronic emotional and/or behavioral symptoms.
   a. Transfer
   b. Discharge
   c. Admission
   d. Adjustment Difficulty
3. An adjustment disorder/stress response syndrome is the same as post-traumatic stress disorder (PTSD). True or **False**
4. A resident's personal property is noted and accounted for on which of the following?
   a. Inventory Sheet
   b. Admission Assessment Sheet
   c. Care Plan Sheet
   d. Nurses notes
5. Personal History should include consideration of which of the following?
   a. Personal history
   b. Personal preferences
   c. Personal routines
   d. All of the above
6. **Postmortem care refers to care at what point?**
   A. After death
   B. Before death
   C. After fall
   D. None of the above

7. Care that focuses on providing comfort and improving quality of life by relieving pain and other symptoms particularly at end of life is known as which of the following?
    a. Postmortem care
    b. Palliative Care
    c. Post-Surgical Care
    d. Pre-Surgical Care
8. Legal document that specifies a person's wishes in regard to withdrawing or withholding life-sustaining procedures and directs the medical treatments a person will accept, or reject is known as which of the following?
    a. Durable Power of Attorney for Health Care
    b. Palliative Plan of Care
    c. Living Will
    d. Hospice Plan of Care
9. A written authorization to represent or act on another's behalf in private affairs, business, or some other legal matter is known as which of the following?
    a. Durable Power of Attorney for Health Care
    b. Palliative Plan of Care
    c. Living Will
    d. Hospice Plan of Care
10. A pattern of breathing in which respirations gradually increase in rate and depth and then become shallow and slow, breathing may stop for 10 to 20 seconds is known as which of the following?
    a. Normal Respirations
    b. Death Rattle
    c. Cheyne-Stoke
    d. None of the above
11. Physical preparation for surgery may include which of the following?
    A. Complete medical history, including medications taken
    B. Lab Work, Chest x-ray or EKG
    C. Bowel Preparation if lower GI surgery
    D. All of the above
12. If a resident is NPO what does that mean?

- **A.** **Nothing by mouth**
- **B.** No perineal care
- **C.** No oral care
- **D.** None of the above

13. Which of the following are potential signs of infection in a surgical site?

- **A.** Redness
- **B.** Odor
- **C.** Swelling
- **D.** **All of the above**

14. What measures might the CNA be asked to assure for the resident following surgery?

- **A.** Take, record and report changes in vital signs
- **B.** Encourage movement and ambulation per doctors' orders.
- C. Monitor for Signs and Symptoms of Infection
- **D.** **All of the above**

15. Post-operative care often includes the following?

- **A.** Wound Care
- **B.** Pain Management
- **C.** **Both A and B**
- D. None of the above

16. An unpleasant sensory and emotional experience associated with actual or potential tissue damage or described in terms of such damage is the definition for which of the following?

- A. Analgesic
- **B.** **Pain**
- C. Nonpharmalogical Intervention
- D. Sensors

17. Which of the following is considered the 5th vital sign?

- **a.** **Pain**
- b. TPR

c. B/P
d. Color

18. When completing a pain scale which would be used for the resident with advanced dementia?
    a. Number Scale
    b. Faces Scale
    c. **PAINAD Scale**
    d. None of the above

19. Heat, Cold, Relaxation Therapy, Aroma Therapy are all examples of which kind of pain intervention?
    a. Pharmacological
    b. **Non-pharmacological**
    c. Specialized Therapy
    d. None of the above

20. Analgesics are an example of which type of intervention.
    a. **Pharmacological**
    b. Non-pharmacological
    c. Specialized Therapy
    d. None of the above

21. A sudden feeling of physical discomfort and distress and is usually the result of an accident, injury or sudden illness (heart attack, appendicitis) describes which of the following?
    a. **Acute Pain**
    b. Chronic Pain
    c. Phantom Pain
    d. None of the above

22. Pain that is ongoing and usually lasts longer than six months is which type of pain?
    a. Acute Pain

b. **Chronic Pain**
c. Phantom Pain
d. None of the above

23. On the pain number scale a score of 8 would indicate what level of pain?
a. Mild
b. Moderate
c. **Severe**
d. Very Severe

24. Barriers are used between the skin and heat or cold application for which of the following reasons?
a. Prevent Infection
b. **Prevent Skin Injury**
c. Prevent Contamination
d. None of the above

25. Process of filtering and removing waste products from the blood used when the kidneys are not functioning properly is known as which of the following?
a. **Dialysis**
b. Hypotension
c. Chronic Kidney Disease
d. Constipation

26. Gradual loss of kidney function over a period of months to years is which of the following?
a. Acute Renal Failure
b. **Chronic Kidney Failure**
c. Venous Catheter
d. Hemodialysis

27. Observation of potential problems of dialysis must be monitored for and reported immediately and include which of the following?
a. **Redness, bleeding or drainage (pus) around the surgical site of catheters**

b. Halitosis
c. Hyperglycemia
d. Apnea

28. Which of the following are potential complications of peritoneal dialysis?

a. Infections.

b. Weight gain.

c. Both A and B

d. None of the above

29. To provide comfort for the resident receiving oxygen therapy the CNA should do which of the following?
A. Ensure the elastic headband is very tight
B. Be sure the face mask is loose
C. Keep skin under mask or cannula clean and dry
D. Wipe face mask out a least once per week.

30. Signs and Symptoms of hypoxia or other respiratory distress include which of the following?
A. Decreased muscle coordination, slowed mental status, and confusion
B. Dyspnea, cyanosis, or pallor
C. Increased rate and depth of respirations
D. All of the above

31. A position assumed to relieve orthopnea is which of the following?
A. Supine
B. Prone
C. Orthopneic position

D. Trendelenburg

32. Which is the most common device used to administer oxygen?

A. Nasal Cannula
B. Simple face mask
C. Partial rebreather mask
D. Venti-mask

33. Frequent oral care should be given to the resident receiving oxygen therapy for which of the following reasons?

A. Oxygen can cause excessive moisture and thrush can grow
B. Oxygen is drying and can dry the oral mucus membranes out.
C. The person receiving oxygen therapy needs oral care like all other residents and does not need any special attention
D. None of the above

34. A resident who breaths primarily through their mouth would need which of the following types of oxygen administration?

A. Simple Face Mask
B. Tracheotomy
C. Respirator
D. Nasal Cannula.

35. Basic tasks that must be accomplished every day for an individual to thrive and include bathing, eating, dressing, etc. are known as which of the following?

A. Independence in Living (IIL)
B. Activities of Daily Living (ADL's)
C. Dependent Care of an Individual
D. Fall Risk Assessment

36. When assessment is completed the intradisciplinary team reviews the information and formulates interventions for the staff to follow. This becomes the document that all staff use to direct care. What is this document?

A. MDS
B. Care Plan
C. Advanced Directive

D. None of the above

37. How the resident moves to and from lying position, turns from side to side, and positions body while in bed or alternative sleep furniture is an assessment of which of the following?

A. **Bed Mobility**
B. Eating
C. Toileting
D. Personal Hygiene

38. How resident uses the toilet room, commode, bedpan, or urinal; transfers on/off toilet; cleans self after elimination; changes pad, manages ostomy or catheter; and adjusts cloths. Do not include emptying of bedpan, urinal, bedside commode, catheter bag or ostomy bag. This is an assessment of which of the following?

A. Bed Mobility
B. Eating
C. **Toileting**
D. Personal Hygiene

39. Individuals with impaired balance and unsteadiness during transitions and walking — are at increased risk for falls and which of the following?

A. often are afraid of falling.
B. may limit their physical and social activity, becoming socially isolated and despondent about limitations.
C. can become increasingly immobile
D. **All of the above**

40. Seating and positioning devices accomplish which of the following:

i. improve body stability,
ii. provide trunk and head support, and
iii. reduce pressure on skin.
iv. **All of the above**

41. Any manual method or physical or mechanical device, material, or equipment attached to or adjacent to the resident's body that the individual cannot remove easily which restricts freedom of movement or normal access to one's body is which of the following?

i. **Physical Restraint**
ii. Chemical Restraint

iii. Safety Device
iv. Mobility Device

42. Any drug used for discipline or convenience and not required to treat medical symptoms is known as which of the following?

A. Physical Restraint
B. Chemical Restraint
C. Safety Device
D. Mobility Device

43. An example of a seating or positioning device would include which of the following?

A. Cane
B. Cushion
C. Walker
D. Wheelchair

44. A broad base of support for body mechanics includes standing with the feet approximately how far apart?

A. Apart about 18" with one foot at right angle to the other
B. Apart about 18" with one foot slightly ahead of the other.
C. As close together as possible no more than 3".
D. As far apart as you can get them so that you can bend when lifting.

45. Which of the following are complications of immobility?

A. Contractures, blood clots, pressure sores or constipation
B. Halitosis,
C. Diaphoresis

46. A discipline of therapy involved in the evaluation, diagnosis, and treatment of communication disorders (speech disorders and language disorders), cognitive-communication disorders, voice disorders, and swallowing disorders is which of the following?

A. Physical Therapy

B. Occupational Therapy
C. **<u>Speech Therapy</u>**
D. Respiratory Therapy

47. Lying the resident/patients' back is said to be in which of the following positions?

A. Trendelenburg
B. **<u>Supine</u>**
C. Prone
D. Lateral or Sims

48. Using correct techniques in performing certain functions in a manner that does not add undue strain to the body is known as which of the following?

A. **<u>Body Mechanics</u>**
B. Body Alignment
C. Positioning
D. Vital signs

49. The resident's position should be changed at least how often?

A. **<u>Every 2 hours or as directed by the care plan</u>**
B. Once per shift
C. Only when they ask to have their position changed
D. At least once in 24 hours

50. The resident uses a cane on which of the following sides?

A. Either side
B. Weaker Side
C. **<u>Strong Side</u>**
D. None of the above

51.To move a joint in a circular motion is which of the following?

A. Pronation
B. Rotation
C. Flexion
D. Hyperextension

52.Which of the following terms describes moving away from the midline of the body?

A. Pronation
B. Rotation
C. Abduction
D. Hyperextension

53.The nurse assistant does the exercise by supporting above and below the joint. The resident is unable to move the joint on their own. Which type of ROM is this?

A. Active
B. Active-Assistive
C. Passive
D. Adduction

54. An ulcer that forms on the skin over a bony area because of pressure is known as which of the following?

A. Pressure Ulcer
B. Stomach Ulcer
C. Diabetic Ulcer
D. None of the above

55.Any point on the body where the bone is immediately below the skin surface is known as which of the following?

A. Bone spur
B. Fracture
C. Bony Prominence
D. Deep Tissue Injury

56. When is the best time to do a head-to-toe skin assessment?

A. Bath Time
B. When setting in the dining room eating
C. During Activities
D. Once a quarter

57. The water for a tub bath should be at which of the following temperatures?
A. 98 degrees F
B. 100 degrees F
C. 105 degrees F
D. 110 degrees F

58. Which of the following are points to remember when performing personal care?
A. Do not allow the resident to assist in the procedures.
B. Gather equipment needed after the procedures start
C. Wash your hands before starting any procedure
D. Personal items can be borrowed from other residents

59. Shaving should be performed in which of the following places?
A. Nurses' station
B. Resident's room or bathroom
C. Clean Utility Room
D. Dining Room

60. Warm water can cause a resident to feel faint. What action should the nurse assistant take if the resident appears faint or says they feel they may faint?

A. Stay with the resident and call for help
B. Drain the tub or shut the water off
C. Lower the head as much as possible and cover the resident with a bath blanket
D. All of the above

61. Powder can be used to help absorb moisture in areas where skin meets skin. The best way to apply powder and not cause caking and further skin irritation includes which of the following?

A. Place directly on the skin and rub back and forth with your fingers
B. Place on a washcloth and use the cloth like a powder puff to lightly dust the area.
C. Shake the powder over the area and get a good coating on the skin.
D. None of the above

62. A condition (found chiefly in women) in which there is involuntary emission of urine when pressure within the abdomen increases suddenly, as in coughing or jumping id which type of incontinence?

A. Urge incontinence
B. Functional incontinence
C. Stress incontinence
D. Overflow incontinence

63. Inability to control the passage of urine is known as which of the following?

A. Constipation
B. Incontinence
C. Impaction
D. None of the above
E. None of the above

64. A pelvic floor exercise that may help with incontinence involves contracting pelvic floor muscles and releasing is known as which of the following?

A. **<u>Kegel Exercise</u>**
B. Abduction
C. Adduction
D. Flexion

65. Residents with incontinence may be at risk for which of the following?
A. Falls
B. Skin Breakdown
C. Pressure ulcers
D. **<u>All of the above</u>**

66. Symptoms include watery diarrhea, fever, nausea, and abdominal pain. It makes up about 20% of cases of antibiotic-associated diarrhea. This describes which of the following?
A. Constipation
B. **<u>CDI or *Clostridioides difficile* infection</u>**
C. Urinary Tract Infection
D. Diverticulosis

67. Surgically created opening that is kept open for drainage or the removal of waste is which of the following?
A. **<u>Stoma</u>**
B. Pouch
C. Rectum
D. None of the above

68. Indigestible fiber of fruits, vegetables, and cereal that acts as a stimulus to aid intestinal peristalsis (e.g., bran, potato skins, fruit skins) is known as which of the following?
A. Minerals
B. **<u>Fiber</u>**
C. Vitamins
D. Proteins

69. Hard stool that cannot pass from the rectum normally is known as which of the following?

A. **Impaction**
B. Diarrhea
C. Fiber
D. Laxative

70. The passage of unusually dry, hard stool is known as which of the following?

A. Impaction
B. Diarrhea
C. **Constipation**
D. Fiber

71. Wavelike movements of the digestive tract that move food through the intestinal tract is known as which of the following?

A. Stoma
B. Ostomy
C. Constipation
D. **Peristalsis**

72. The small passage from the bladder through which urine leaves the body is known as which of the following?

A. **Urethra**
B. Bladder
C. Ureter
D. Kidney

73. Cleansing the genital and anal area of the resident is known as which of the following?

A. **Perineal Care**
B. Bladder Care
C. Bowel Care
D. Catheter Care

74. A sterile tube inserted through the urethra into the bladder to drain urine; held in place by a small, inflated balloon is which of the following?

A. IV

B. Pic Line

C. **Indwelling urinary catheter (foley)**

D. Cannula

75. Loose skin at and covering the end of the penis on uncircumcised males is known as which of the following?

A. **Foreskin**

B. Penial tip

C. Urethra

D. Scrotum

76. Inability to empty the bladder is known as which of the following?

A. Incontinence

B. **Retention**

C. Continence

D. Nocturia

77. When performing perineal care, the CNA should do which of the following to prevent potential infection?

A. Wipe from back to front

B. **Wipe from front to back**

C. Clean from dirtiest to cleanest

D. None of the above

78. How often should a resident who is comatose, NPO or receiving oxygen have oral care?

A. Every shift

B. After each meal

C. **Every Two Hours**

D. It is not necessary since they are not eating

79. Which of the following are reasons to perform oral care on comatose, NPO or residents receiving oxygen?

A. Stick substances can build up in the mouth
B. Mouth breathing and oxygen use can be drying to the mouth
C. Both A and B
D. None of the above

80. When performing oral care on a comatose resident the head should be in which of the following positions to prevent choking?
    A. **To the Side**
    B. Straight Back resting on the back of the head
    C. Tilted forward chin down
    D. It doesn't really matter which position the head is in

81. Dentures are expensive. When brushing dentures what should be placed in the bottom of the sink as cushion in case they are dropped?
    A. Water is sufficient
    B. **A washcloth on the bottom covered with 3-4 inches of water**
    C. Foam cushions
    D. None of the above

82. Oral care should be provided how often for all residents?
    A. Once per day
    B. Once per shift
    C. **Twice per day**
    D. At least weekly

83. Special diet used as a treatment for a disease or condition is known as which of the following?
    A. Micronutrient
    B. Macronutrient
    C. **Therapeutic Diet**
    D. Nutrient

84. The resident drank an 8-ounce cup of coffee this morning for breakfast. How many cc is that fluid intake?

A. 30 cc intake
B. 90 cc intake
C. 240 cc intake
D. 360 cc intake

85. The resident toileted 3 times on your shift. The first you measured 120 cc of urine, the second you measured 200 cc of urine and the third you measured 180 cc of urine. How many cc of urine output did the resident have on your shift?
A. 480 cc output
B. 500 cc output
C. 320 cc output
D. 580 cc output

86. Supplying water to the body to maintain fluid balance is known as which of the following?
A. Dehydration
B. Hydration
C. Malnutrition
D. Dysphagia

87. The medical term for difficulty swallowing is which of the following?
A. Dehydration
B. Hydration
C. Malnutrition
D. Dysphagia

88. Which of the following would be normal fluid intake for an adult older resident?
A. Between 500 and 1000 cc per 24 hours
B. Between 1500 and 2000 cc per 24 hours
C. Less than 1200 cc per 24 hours
D. More than 3000 cc per 24 hours

89. Normal urine output for a resident is which of the following?

A. Approximately 800 cc per 24 hours

B. More than 2000 cc per 24 hours

C. **About 1500 cc per 24 hours**

D. None of the above

90. An infection that residents acquire, that is associated with a medical or surgical intervention (e.g., podiatry, wound care debridement) within a nursing home and was not present or incubating at the time of admission. Is which of the following?

A. MRSA

B. **Healthcare Acquired Infection (HAI)**

C. MDRO

D. Parasite

91. Sudden increase in cases of a disease within a certain geographic area or within a facility, school, community, etc. is known as which of the following?

A. **Outbreak**

B. HAI

C. MDRO

D. MRSA

92. The second tier of basic infection control and is to be used in addition to Standard Precautions for patients who may be infected or colonized with certain infectious agents for which additional precautions are needed to prevent infection transmission describes which of the following?

A. Isolation

B. Standard Precautions

C. **Transmission Based Precautions**

D. None of the Above

93. The three categories of Transmission-Based Precautions include:

A. Contact Precautions,
B. Droplet Precautions,
C. Airborne Precautions.
D. <u>All of the above</u>

94. The use of which of the transmission-based precautions applies when respiratory droplets contain viruses or bacteria particles which may be spread to another susceptible individual?

A. Contact Precautions,
B. **<u>Droplet Precautions</u>**,
C. Airborne Precautions.
D. All the above

95. This transmission-based precaution is intended to prevent transmission of infections that are spread by direct (e.g., person-to-person) or indirect contact with the resident or environment, and require the use of appropriate PPE, including a gown and gloves upon entering (i.e., before making contact with the resident or resident's environment) the room or cubicle. Prior to leaving the resident's room or cubicle, the PPE is removed, and hand hygiene is performed.

A. <u>Contact Precautions,</u>
B. Droplet Precautions,
C. Airborne Precautions.
D. All of the above

96. Which of the following are necessary for an infection to occur?

A. Source: Places where infectious agents (germs) live (e.g., sinks, surfaces, human skin)
B. Susceptible Person with a way for germs to enter the body
C. Transmission: a way germ(s) is moved to the susceptible person
D. **<u>All the above</u>**

97. Covering the mouth and nose with a tissue when coughing or sneezing and disposing of the used tissue in the nearest waste receptacle are examples of which of the following?
    - **A. Respiratory Hygiene or Etiquette**
    - **B.** Respiratory Isolation
    - C. Methods to prevent urinary tract infections
    - D. None of the above
98. When should gloves be used when providing direct patient care?
    - A. All times regardless of what you are doing
    - B. Any time that you will touch the resident, even on the hand
    - **C. When there is potential contact with blood, body fluids, secretion or excretion.**
    - D. Handwashing is enough gloves are only necessary when cleaning with chemicals.
99. Handwashing should occur before which of the following?
    - A. Resident/Patient Contact
    - B. Handling Food
    - C. Starting your shift
    - **D. All the above**

100. Specialized clothing or equipment worn by an employee for protection against infectious materials is known as which of the following?
    - **A.** Isolation Dress
    - **B. Personal Protective Equipment**
    - C. Hand Hygiene
    - D. Transmission

Becoming a Certified Nurse Assistant: A Person-Centered Approach

Take Oral Temperature

Competency Sheet: Unit III, LP 4

Name of Student: ______________________________

Equipment Needed:

Glass Oral Thermometer or Electronic thermometer and probe cover (disposable)
Watch with second hand
Alcohol swabs and tissue
Chart or form for recording
Pen and Paper
Gloves (if there is a possibility of contact with body fluids)

The Student Completed the Following	Yes	No
1. Gathered the necessary equipment		
2. Identify and greet the resident. Identify Self		
3. Wash your hands. Glove if needed.		
4. Wash your hands. Glove if needed.		
5. Provide privacy.		
6. Ask the resident if they've eaten or drank anything or smoked in the last five minutes. If so wait at least 15 minutes.		
7. Using a glass bulb thermometer a. Rinse thermometer if it has been soaked in disinfectant solution.		
b. Check thermometer for any cracks or chips (if found do not use-get another)		
c. Shake the thermometer down to 94 F or below (firmly grasp the stem end and snap your wrist several times until achieved degree is reached)		
d. Ask the resident to open mouth and raise tongue. Place the thermometer bulb under the resident's tongue toward the side of the mouth.		
e. Instruct the resident to hold the bulb end under the tongue and hold in place by closing his/her lips around the thermometer. Leave in place for 5 minutes. (Remind not to talk)		
f. Grasp the stem end of the thermometer and remove it from the resident's mouth and wipe with a tissue toward the bulb from the stem.		
g. Read the thermometer.		
h. Record the temperature reading on the paper or the kiosk for the EHR system or both.		
i. Shake down the thermometer.		
j. Disinfect with alcohol swab or return to disinfectant		
8. Using an electronic Thermometer a. Disinfect the electronic thermometer by using alcohol swab to swipe entire surface.		

b. Make sure the oral probe is plugged into the thermometer.		
c. Remove probe from unit and insert it into a probe cover (disposable)		
d. Ask resident to open mouth and raise tongue; place covered probe at the base of the tongue on either side of the mouth.		
e. Ask resident to lower tongue and close mouth.		
f. Hold the probe in the resident's mouth until the tone is heard or when there is a flashing or steady light.		
g. Read the temperature reading on the digital display.		
h. Remove the covered probe and dispose of the cover by pressing the eject button.		
i. Record the temperature reading on paper and/or EHR Kiosk		
j. Return the probe to the holder.		
k. Use Alcohol Swab to disinfect all surfaces on the probe		
9. Remove gloves, if used and dispose of appropriately. Wash hands.		
10. Make resident comfortable and place call signal within reach.		
11. Remove, clean and store equipment. Place glass thermometer in disinfectant or follow facility policy and procedure.		
12. Record observations and report anything unusual to the charge nurse.		

The student/employee has satisfactorily completed the procedure and demonstrated competency for the skill: "**Take an Oral Temperature**" according to the steps outlined. Ask the student/employee questions about the procedure to assure they understand the process and what the information is used for.

____ __________________

Instructor/Clinical Supervisor Signature Date

Becoming a Certified Nurse Assistant: A Person-Centered Approach

Take Rectal Temperature

Competency Sheet: Unit III, LP 4

Name of Student: ____

Equipment Needed:

Glass Rectal Thermometer or Electronic thermometer (do not use same device for rectal that you do for oral) and probe cover (disposable)

Watch with secondhand
Pen and Paper
Water-soluble lubricant
Chart or form for recording
Gloves
Alcohol swabs and tissue

The Student Completed the Following	Yes	No
1. Gathered the necessary equipment		
2. Identify and greet the resident. Identify Self		
3. Wash your hands.		
4. Glove		
5. Provide privacy.		
6. Ask the resident if they've had recent diarrhea or have any rectal issues. If so check with charge nurse before proceeding.		
7. Using a glass bulb thermometer a. Rinse thermometer if it has been soaked in disinfectant solution.		
b. Check thermometer for any cracks or chips (if found do not use-get another)		
c. Shake the thermometer down to 94 F or below (firmly grasp the stem end and snap your wrist several times until achieved degree is reached)		
d. Instruct the resident to lie on their side with upper leg flexed.		
e. Put a small amount of lubricant on a tissue and lubricate the bulb end of the thermometer		
f. Raise the upper buttock to expose the anus; insert the bulb end of the thermometer 1 inch into the rectum. Cover the resident but do not let go of the thermometer.		
g. Hold thermometer in place 3 to 4 minutes while holding the top hip of the resident to prevent them from rolling back.		
h. Remove the thermometer. Wipe it clean with the tissue from the stem to the bulb.		
i. Place the thermometer on a clean toilet tissue; wipe the anal area to remove excess lubricant.		
j. Cover the resident		
k. Read the thermometer and record on paper and/or EHR the temperature reading.		
l. Shake down the thermometer		
m. Remove, store and clean equipment. Disinfect glass thermometer.		

n. Remove gloves and dispose in appropriate container, wash hands.		
8. Using an electronic Thermometer a. Disinfect the electronic thermometer by using alcohol swab to swipe entire surface.		
b. Make sure the rectal probe is plugged into the thermometer. (rectal probe is usually red)		
c. Remove probe from unit and insert it into a probe cover (disposable)		
d. Ask resident to lie on side with upper leg flexed.		
e. Lubricate the probe cover.		
f. Raise the upper buttock to expose the anus; insert the probe 1 inch into the rectum. Cover the resident but do not let go of the thermometer.		
g. Hold the thermometer until a tone is heard or when there is a flashing or steady light.		
h. Read the temperature on the digital display.		
i. Remove the covered probe and dispose of the cover by pressing the eject button.		
j. Record the temperature reading on paper and/or EHR Kiosk		
k. Return the probe to the holder.		
l. Use Alcohol Swab to disinfect all surfaces on the probe		
m. Cover the resident.		
9. Remove gloves, if used and dispose of appropriately. Wash hands.		
10. Make resident comfortable and place call signal within reach.		
11. Remove, clean and store equipment. Place glass thermometer in disinfectant or follow facility policy and procedure.		
12. Record observations and report anything unusual to the charge nurse.		

The student/employee has satisfactorily completed the procedure and demonstrated competency for the skill: "**Take a Rectal Temperature**" according to the steps outlined. Ask the student/employee questions about the procedure to assure they understand the process and what the information is used for.

______________________________ ____________________

Instructor/Clinical Supervisor Signature Date

Becoming a Certified Nurse Assistant: A Person-Centered Approach

Take Tympanic Artery (forehead) Temperature

Competency Sheet: Unit III, LP 4

Name of Student: ______________________________

Equipment Needed:

Tympanic forehead Thermometer (electronic) with disposable probe cover
Alcohol swabs
Pen and Paper
Chart or form for recording

The Student Completed the Following	Yes	No
1. Gathered the necessary equipment		
2. Identify and greet the resident. Identify Self		
3. Wash your hands.		
4. Explain what you are going to do.		
5. Provide privacy.		
6. <u>Using a Tympanic Artery (forehead) Thermometer</u> a. Disinfect the thermometer by using alcohol swab to swipe entire surface.		
b. Remove hair and any other coverings away from forehead.		
c. Cover the probe with a disposable cover		
d. Hold the "on" button and place the probe on the center of the forehead. Still holding the "on" button, slide the probe, horizontally, across the forehead to the hairline.		
e. With the "on" button still pressed, place the probe on the neck, behind the ear lobe.		
f. Release the "on" button and read the digital temperature results.		
g. Discard the plastic cover by pushing the eject button.		
h. Record results on paper and/or EHR		
i. Remove, store and clean equipment.		
j. Disinfect the electronic thermometer by using alcohol swab to swipe entire surface.		
7. Wash hands.		
8. Make resident comfortable and place call signal within reach.		
9. Remove, clean and store equipment.		

10. Record observations and report anything unusual to the charge nurse.		

The student/employee has satisfactorily completed the procedure and demonstrated competency for the skill: "**Take a Tympanic Artery (forehead)Temperature**" according to the steps outlined. Ask the student/employee questions about the procedure to assure they understand the process and what the information is used for.

_______________________________ _______________________________

Instructor/Clinical Supervisor Signature Date

Becoming a Certified Nurse Assistant: A Person-Centered Approach

Take Tympanic Temperature

Competency Sheet: Unit III, LP 4

Name of Student: ______________________________

Equipment Needed:

Tympanic Thermometer (electronic)
Alcohol swabs
Chart or form for recording
Pen and Paper
Gloves (if needed such as drainage from the ear)

The Student Completed the Following	Yes	No
1. Gathered the necessary equipment		
2. Identify and greet the resident. Identify Self		
3. Wash your hands.		
4. Explain what you are going to do.		
5. Provide privacy.		
6. <u>Using a Tympanic Thermometer</u> a. Instruct the resident to turn their head to one side to easily access the ear.		
b.		
c. If there is visible ear wax in the ear canal opening, wipe away access from the other ear canal only. Do not wipe into the inner ear.		
d. Remove the thermometer from the charger		
e. Cover the speculum (the probe end) with a disposable cover.		
f. Gently pull the ear up and back for adults or straight back for children and then insert the speculum.		
g. Remove the probe when you hear a beep..		
h. Discard the plastic speculum cover by pushing the eject button.		
i. Read the thermometer and record on paper and/or EHR the temperature reading.		
j. Remove, store and clean equipment.		
k. Remove gloves (if used) and dispose in appropriate container, wash hands.		
l. Disinfect the electronic thermometer by using alcohol swab to swipe entire surface.		
m. Read the temperature on the digital display.		
7. Remove gloves, if used and dispose of appropriately. Wash hands.		
8. Make resident comfortable and place call signal within reach.		

9. Remove, clean and store equipment.		
10. Record observations and report anything unusual to the charge nurse.		

The student/employee has satisfactorily completed the procedure and demonstrated competency for the skill: "**Take a Tympanic Temperature**" according to the steps outlined. Ask the student/employee questions about the procedure to assure they understand the process and what the information is used for.

_________________________________ _________________

Instructor/Clinical Supervisor Signature Date

Take Radial Pulse

Competency Sheet: Unit III, LP 4

Name of Student: ____

Equipment Needed:

Watch with second hand
Chart or form for recording
Pen and Paper

The Student Completed the Following	Yes	No
1. Gathered the necessary equipment		
2. Identify and greet the resident. Identify Self		
3. Wash your hands.		
4. Explain what you are going to do.		
5. Provide privacy.		
6. Resident should be in a sitting or supine position.		
7. Locate radial pulse with your fingertips (do not use thumb)		
8. Note the rhythm and the force of the pulse		
9. Count the pulse for 1 full minute. If you are unsure check and count again.		
10. Note any abnormal characteristics of the pulse		
11. Record results on paper and/or EHR		
12. Wash hands.		
13. Make resident comfortable and place call signal within reach.		
14. Remove, clean and store equipment.		
15. Record observations and report anything unusual to the charge nurse.		

The student/employee has satisfactorily completed the procedure and demonstrated competency for the skill: "**Take Radial Pulse**" according to the steps outlined. Ask the student/employee questions about the procedure to assure they understand the process and what the information is used for.

____ ________________________

Instructor/Clinical Supervisor Signature Date

Becoming a Certified Nurse Assistant: A Person-Centered Approach

Take Apical Pulse

Competency Sheet: Unit III, LP 4

Name of Student: ______________________________

Equipment Needed:

Watch with secondhand
Alcohol swabs
Stethoscope with diaphragm
Chart or form for recording
Pen and Paper

The Student Completed the Following	Yes	No
1. Gathered the necessary equipment		
2. Identify and greet the resident. Identify Self		
3. Wash your hands.		
4. Explain what you are going to do.		
5. Provide privacy.		
6. Resident should be in a sitting or supine position.		
7. Clean the earpieces and diaphragm with alcohol wipes		
8. Raise the resident's gown or upper clothing to expose the nipple are of the left chest. Do not expose more of the chest than is necessary.		
9. Warm the diaphragm of the stethoscope with your hands		
10. Place the earpieces in your ears		
11. Locate the apical pulse. The diaphragm should be placed just below the left nipple.		
12. Listen carefully.		
13. Count the pulse for 1 full minute. Note if the pulse is regular or irregular.		
14. Record results on paper and/or EHR		
15. Wash hands.		
16. Cover the resident		
17. Make resident comfortable and place call signal within reach.		
18. Remove, clean and store equipment. (Clean earpieces and diaphragm with alcohol swabs.		
19. Record observations and report anything unusual to the charge nurse.		

The student/employee has satisfactorily completed the procedure and demonstrated competency for the skill: "**Take Apical Pulse**" according to the steps outlined. Ask the student/employee questions about the procedure to assure they understand the process and what the information is used for.

______________________________ ______________________________

Instructor/Clinical Supervisor Signature Date

Becoming a Certified Nurse Assistant: A Person-Centered Approach

Count Respirations

Competency Sheet: Unit III, LP 4

Name of Student: ______________________________

Equipment Needed:

Watch with secondhand   Pen and Paper

Chart or form for recording

The Student Completed the Following	Yes	No
1. Gathered the necessary equipment		
2. Identify and greet the resident. Identify Self		
3. Wash your hands.		
4. Explain what you are going to do.		
5. Provide privacy.		
6. Resident should be in a sitting or supine position.		
7. Rest resident's arms across his/her chest with your fingers on radial pulse for ease in observing rise and fall of chest cavity during respirations		
8. Begin counting respirations when you see the chest rise; count respirations for 1 full minute. Recount if unsure.		
9. Note any abnormal characteristics of respirations		
10. Record results on paper and/or EHR		
11. Wash hands.		
12. Make resident comfortable and place call signal within reach.		
13. Record observations and report anything unusual to the charge nurse.		

The student/employee has satisfactorily completed the procedure and demonstrated competency for the skill: **"Count Respirations"** according to the steps outlined. Ask the student/employee questions about the procedure to assure they understand the process and what the information is used for.

______________________________   ____________________

Instructor/Clinical Supervisor Signature   Date

Measure Blood Pressure

Competency Sheet: Unit III, LP 4

Name of Student: ______________________________

Equipment Needed:

Sphygmomanometer
Stethoscope
Alcohol Sponges
Chart or form for recording
Pen and Paper

The Student Completed the Following	Yes	No
1. Gathered the necessary equipment		
2. Identify and greet the resident. Identify Self		
3. Wash your hands.		
4. Explain what you are going to do.		
5. Provide privacy.		
6. Resident should be in a sitting or supine position. Position the entire lower arm on a flat surface palm upward		
7. Clean the earpieces and diaphragm of the stethoscope with alcohol swabs.		
8. Expose the arm as much as possible. Squeeze cuff to expel any remaining air and turn valve clockwise on the bulb to close it. Note: Careful not to tighten it too much or you might have trouble opening it.		
9. Wrap cuff around the upper with the bottom edge about 1" above the elbow. The rubber tubing should come out toward the hand. Be sure the cuff is the appropriate size. Center the bladder (bag inside the cuff) over the brachial artery. (some cuffs are marked with arrow)		
10. Locate the brachial pulse at the inner aspect of the elbow with your fingers and place the diaphragm over the brachial (artery) the pulse site (Again, don't use your thumb). Do not stuff the diaphragm of the stethoscope under the cuff. It can be painful and distort the reading.		
11. Place the earpieces of the stethoscope in your ears		
12. Hold the rubber bulb in your hand (the one not holding the stethoscope)		
13. Quickly inflate the cuff with air by pumping the bulb. Watch the gauge and pump to 170-200 mm Hg.		
14. Slightly loosen the valve counterclockwise. Deflate slowly and steadily while you listen carefully. Watch the gauge for the first time you hear the beat of the heart through the artery. This is the systolic reading, or the top number Note that number in your mind. Continue to listen until you no longer hear the pulse beat. At the last sound on the gauge this is the diastolic pressure (lower number). Note: If you immediately hear pulse sounds, stop procedure, delete and remove cuff. Wait 15 seconds and then reapply cuff and repeat inflating the cuff to a higher caliber of 200-220 mm Hg. If pulse sounds at 220 mm Hg immediately stop and report to the charge nurse.		
15. Deflate the cuff, remove earpieces from your ears, remove cuff from the resident's arm and squeeze excess air out of the cuff.		

16. Record results on paper and/or EHR		
17. Wash hands.		
18. Make resident comfortable and place call signal within reach.		
19. Clean and store equipment. Disinfect the stethoscope with alcohol swabs (earpieces and diaphragm).		
20. Record observations and report anything unusual to the charge nurse.		

The student/employee has satisfactorily completed the procedure and demonstrated competency for the skill: "**Measure Blood Pressure"** according to the steps outlined. Ask the student/employee questions about the procedure to assure they understand the process and what the information is used for.

__________________________________ ______________________

Instructor/Clinical Supervisor Signature Date

Becoming a Certified Nurse Assistant: A Person-Centered Approach

Measure Pulse Oximetry

Competency Sheet: Unit III, LP 4

Equipment Name of Student: ______________________________

Needed:

Pulse Oximetry Device   Chart or form for recording
Alcohol Sponges   Pen and Paper

The Student Completed the Following	Yes	No
1. Gathered the necessary equipment		
2. Identify and greet the resident. Identify Self		
3. Wash your hands.		
4. Explain what you are going to do.		
5. Provide privacy.		
6. Resident should be in a sitting or supine position. Position the entire lower arm on a flat surface palm upward		
7. Clean the pulse oximetry device with alcohol swabs to disinfect.		
8. Expose a finger on either hand. And apply the sensor to the finger.		
9. Turn pulse oximetry on and wait for beep or fixed digital readout to appear.		
10. Record results on paper and/or EHR		
11. Wash hands.		
12. Make resident comfortable and place call signal within reach.		
13. Clean and store equipment. Disinfect the pulse oximetry device with alcohol swabs.		
14. Record observations and report anything unusual to the charge nurse.		

The student/employee has satisfactorily completed the procedure and demonstrated competency for the skill: "**Measure Pulse Oximetry"** according to the steps outlined. Ask the student/employee questions about the procedure to assure they understand the process and what the information is used for.

____   ________________

Instructor/Clinical Supervisor Signature   Date

Handwashing

Competency Sheet: Unit VII. LP 1

Name of Student: ____

Equipment Needed:

Water
Soap
Paper Towels
Waste Basket

The Student Completed the Following	Yes	No
1. Remove wristwatch and/or rings. Roll up your sleeves. (wash wristwatch and rings if they have come into contact with contaminated materials)		
2. Turn water on, adjust temperature for comfort. DO NOT TOUCH FAUCETS OR CONTROLS DURING THE REST OF THE PROCEDURE		
3. Wet hands thoroughly, including 2 to 3 inches above the wrists. Hold hands with hands lower than wrists and wrists lower than elbows. Fingertips pointed downward.		
4. Apply a generous amount of soap to hands. DO NOT USE BAR SOAP.		
5. Scrub hands for at least 15 seconds.		
a. Wash palms and back of hands with at least 10 circular motions.		
b. Wash fingers and between fingers with at least 10 circular motions.		
c. Wash wrists with at least 10 circular motions		
d. Wash around and under fingernails.		
6. Rinse wrists and hands well. Keep wrists below elbows with fingers pointing down so that the water drains away from your hands.		
7. Dry hands well with paper towel. Use a clean/new one for each hand.		
8. Take a clean paper towel and shut off faucet. DO NOT TOUCH THE SINK AREA WITH CLEAN HANDS		
9. Discard paper towels in wastebasket being careful not to touch parts of the towel that touched the faucet.		
10. Use a clean paper towel to turn the knob on the door or pull the door open.		

The student/employee has satisfactorily completed the procedure and demonstrated competency for the skill: "**Handwashing**" according to the steps outlined. Ask the student/employee questions about the procedure to assure they understand the process and what the information is used for.

____ ______________________________

Instructor/Clinical Supervisor Signature Date

Becoming a Certified Nurse Assistant: A Person-Centered Approach

Don and Remove Disposable Gloves

Competency Sheet: Unit VII. LP 1

Name of Student: ____

Equipment Needed:

Water
Soap
Paper Towels
Wastebasket
Non-Sterile Gloves

The Student Completed the Following	Yes	No
Put on Gloves		
1. Wash and Dry Hands		
2. Remove gloves from box, one at a time.		
3. Place your hand through the opening and pull the glove up to the wrist		
4. Repeat with the second glove.		
5. Adjust gloves to cover your wrists or cuffs of gown (if wearing). CAUTION: DO NOT TOUCH ANY PART OF YOUR BODY WITH GLOVED HANDS.		
6. Complete Resident Care		
Remove Gloves		
1. Grasp one glove on the inside of the wrist at ½ inch below band of dirty side of glove without touching your skin.		
2. Pull down glove, turning it inside out, and pull off hand. Hold the glove with the still gloved hand.		
3. Insert fingers of ungloved hand under the cuff of the glove on the other hand (on inside of cuff).		
4. Take a clean paper towel and shut off faucet. DO NOT TOUCH THE SINK AREA WITH CLEAN HANDS		
5. Pull down glove until it is inside out, drawing it over the first glove.		
6. Discard both gloves in wastebasket.		
7. Wash hands.		

The student/employee has satisfactorily completed the procedure and demonstrated competency for the skill: "**DON and Remove Disposable Gloves"** according to the steps outlined. Ask the student/employee questions about the procedure to assure they understand the process and what the information is used for.

____ __________

Instructor/Clinical Supervisor Signature Date

Don and Remove Mask

Competency Sheet: Unit VII. LP 1

Name of Student: ________________________________

Equipment Needed:

Water | Mask

Soap

The Student Completed the Following	Yes	No
Put on Gloves		
1. Wash and Dry Hands		
2. Pick up Mask		
3. Adjust mask over nose and mouth		
4. Tie the top string behind head or adjust elastic band		
5. Tie the bottom string behind head or adjust elastic band.		
6. Complete Resident Care (REPLACE MASK IF IT BECOMES MOIST)		
Remove Gloves		
1. Wash hands after removing gloves if worn.		
2. Untie bottom string ore remove elastic band		
3. Untie top string or remove elastic band		
4. Remove by holding top strings		
5. Discard by dropping mask in wastebasket.		
6. Wash hands.		

The student/employee has satisfactorily completed the procedure and demonstrated competency for the skill: **"DON and Remove Mask"** according to the steps outlined. Ask the student/employee questions about the procedure to assure they understand the process and what the information is used for.

________________________________ ____________

Instructor/Clinical Supervisor Signature Date

Don and Remove Nonsterile Gown

Competency Sheet: Unit VII. LP 1

Becoming a Certified Nurse Assistant: A Person-Centered Approach

Name of Student: ______________________________

Equipment Needed:

Water
Soap
Mask (optional)
Paper Towels
Gown
Gloves (Optional)

The Student Completed the Following	Yes	No
Put on Gown		
1. Wash and Dry Hands		
2. Put on Mask if using		
3. Unfold gown with opening at the back		
4. Put on gown by slipping arms into the sleeves		
5. Slip fingers inside the neckband		
6. Tie necktie or fasten strips in back		
7. Grasp waist ties in front and bring to back		
8. Reach behind and overlap edges of gown		
9. Put on gloves		
10. Complete Patient Care		
Remove Gloves		
1. Untie or unfasten waist tie		
2. Remove gloves		
3. Wash Hands		
4. If wearing mask remove		
5. Untie ties or fasteners at neck and loosen gown at neck		
6. Slip fingers of one hand inside the cuff of the other hand (DO NOT TOUCH OUTSIDE OF GOWN)		
7. Pull down gown over hand.		
8. With gown-covered hand, pull down gown over the hand		
9. Fold gown away from your body with contaminated side inward		
10. Wash Hands		
11. If using transmission-based precautions, open door with paper towel. Use to to keep door open while discarding towel in trash receptacle before leaving the resident		
12. Wash hands		

Becoming a Certified Nurse Assistant: A Person-Centered Approach

The student/employee has satisfactorily completed the procedure and demonstrated competency for the skill: "**DON and Remove Nonsterile Gown"** according to the steps outlined. Ask the student/employee questions about the procedure to assure they understand the process and what the information is used for.

____ __________

Instructor/Clinical Supervisor Signature Date

Feeding a Resident

Competency Sheet: Unit VIII. LP 1

Name of Student: ______________________________________

Equipment Needed:

Food Tray
Overbed Table
Napkins or towel
Chair

The Student Completed the Following	Yes	No
1. Wash hands		
2. Perform before-meal care; offer bedpan/urinal, wash resident's hands and face, position the resident in full upright and sitting position.		
3. Wash Hands		
4. Check the food tray with the dietary card and identify the resident to make sure it is correct		
5. Serve one tray at a time to avoid contamination		
6. Serve trays promptly so food temperature is maintained		
7. Carry the tray at waist level not on the shoulders or next to hair		
8. See that the appearance of the tray is orderly and contains utensils, napkins, condiments as allowed		
9. IF the resident requires assistive feeding devices make sure it is on the tray a. Note some facilities practice taking the food items, plates, cups, etc. off the tray and setting them on the table.		
10. Assist in food preparation as needed, open milk cartons, condiments, assist with cutting food up if necessary		
11. Encourage independence and the resident to do as much as possible.		
12. Explain that you will assist the resident to eat		
13. Place napkin, towel or clothing protector, depending on facility policy across chest to protect cloths		
14. Sit down in chair facing resident		
15. Identify what is on the tray and ask what the resident would like first. Remember always try to encourage a drink before starting		
16. Use spoon to give small bites allow time for chewing and swallowing, alternate bites with liquids		
17. Wipe mouth as needed		
18. Warn when offering hot or warm foods		
19. Remove the tray when resident has finished eating. Note the foods and amounts eaten. Ask if there is anything else you could get for the resident,		
20. Offer post-meal care, wash resident's hands and face, remove and discard napkin. If in bed reposition and make sure call light is within reach		
21. Wash hands.		

Becoming a Certified Nurse Assistant: A Person-Centered Approach

The student/employee has satisfactorily completed the procedure and demonstrated competency for the skill: "**Feeding a Resident**" according to the steps outlined. Ask the student/employee questions about the procedure to assure they understand the process and what the information is used for.

____ ___________

Instructor/Clinical Supervisor Signature Date

Serving A Food Tray

Competency Sheet: Unit VIII. LP 1

Name of Student: ______________________________

Equipment Needed:

Food Tray Overbed Table

Napkins or towel Chair

The Student Completed the Following	Yes	No
1. Wash hands		
2. Check the food tray with the dietary card and identify the resident to make sure it is correct		
3. Serve one tray at a time to avoid contamination		
4. Serve trays promptly so food temperature is maintained		
5. Carry the tray at waist level not on the shoulders or next to hair		
6. See that the appearance of the tray is orderly and contains utensils, napkins, condiments as allowed		
7. IF the resident requires assistive feeding devices make sure it is on the tray a. Note some facilities practice taking the food items, plates, cups, etc. off the tray and setting them on the table.		
8. Assist in food preparation as needed, open milk cartons, condiments, assist with cutting food up if necessary		
9. Encourage independence and the resident to do as much as possible.		
10. Remove the tray when resident has finished eating. Note the foods and amounts eaten. Ask if there is anything else you could get for the resident,		
11. Wash hands.		

The student/employee has satisfactorily completed the procedure and demonstrated competency for the skill: "**Serving a Food Tray"** according to the steps outlined. Ask the student/employee questions about the procedure to assure they understand the process and what the information is used for.

______________________________ __________

Instructor/Clinical Supervisor Signature Date

Becoming a Certified Nurse Assistant: A Person-Centered Approach

Perform First Aid for Choking-Conscious Sitting/Standing

Competency Sheet: Unit VI, LP 1

Name of Student: ______________________________

The Student Completed the Following	Yes	No
1. Call for help as you approach the resident. Instruct a coworker to call the charge nurse. Notify 911 or EMS per facility policy.		
2. Explain to the resident that you are going to help		
3. Ask if conscious "Are you choking?" If airway is obstructed resident will not be able to answer.		
4. Position yourself behind the resident		
5. Slide your arms under resident's arms, wrapping both of your arms around the resident's waist		
6. Make a fist and place thumb side of this fist against the midline of the resident's abdomen, just above the navel. Keep the fist below the resident's rib cage and avoid the sternum.		
7. Grasp your fist with your free hand.		
8. Apply pressure and thrust inward and upward		
9. Deliver these inward, upward thrusts until object is dislodged or resident becomes unconscious.		
10. If the resident becomes unconscious assist to a lying position and perform first aid for choking for the unconscious		
11. Continue the thrusts until the object is cleared or medical support arrives.		
12. Record observations and the action you took.		

The student/employee has satisfactorily completed the procedure and demonstrated competency for the skill: "**Perform First Aid for Choking-Conscious Setting or Standing"** according to the steps outlined. Ask the student/employee questions about the procedure to assure they understand the process and what the information is used for.

______________________________ ____________

Instructor/Clinical Supervisor Signature Date

Becoming a Certified Nurse Assistant: A Person-Centered Approach

Perform First Aid for Choking-Unconscious

Competency Sheet: Unit VI, LP 1

Name of Student: ________________________________

The Student Completed the Following	Yes	No
1. Call for help as you approach the resident. Instruct a coworker to call the charge nurse. Notify 911 or EMS per facility policy.		
2. Check for unresponsiveness and no breathing.		
3. Turn resident on his/her back.		
4. Put on gloves		
5. Open airway by tipping the head back and lifting the jaw (head tilt/chin lift maneuver) designed to open the airway. Look, listen and feel for breathing.		
6. With resident's face up, open mouth and grasp tongue and jaw between thumb and index finger, draw tongue forward and do not let the mouth close.		
7. Insert index finger of the other hand down along the side of the cheek toward the base of the tongue.		
8. Sweep around the mouth. Bend finger into hook and attempt to bring foreign object up into the mouth if you can see it. **<u>Caution do not fore objects further into the throat.</u>**		
9. If possible, remove object from the mouth.		
10. Insert mouthpiece if available. Otherwise attempt breathing (one breath every 5 seconds) . Attempt to give two breaths.		
11. If unsuccessful, reposition and reopen airway.		
12. Insert mouthpiece if available and attempt breathing.		
13. If efforts to ventilate are unsuccessful, provide abdominal thrusts five times. Straddle the resident at the level of the hips. Position the heel of one hand on the resident's abdomen at the midline between the navel and rib cage. Note: Fingers should point toward the resident's chest. Keep hand below resident's rib cage, avoiding the area just below the sternum. Place free hand over the positioned hand and put your shoulders directly over the resident's abdomen. Press hands inward and toward the resident's		

diaphragm, as if you are trying to push toward the resident's back. Again give 5 thrusts.		
14. Check the mouth again for foreign objects and remove if possible following steps 5-9 above.		
15. Reopen airway, insert mouthpiece if available and attempt breathing.		
16. Repeat procedures until airway is clear and/or life support is available.		
17. If resident begins breathing remove the mouthpiece and place on left side.		
18. Remove gloves and discard in appropriate container. Wash hands.		
19. Record observations and the action you took.		

The student/employee has satisfactorily completed the procedure and demonstrated competency for the skill: "**Perform First Aid for Choking-Unconscious"** according to the steps outlined. Ask the student/employee questions about the procedure to assure they understand the process and what the information is used for.

____________________________________ __________

Instructor/Clinical Supervisor Signature Date

Becoming a Certified Nurse Assistant: A Person-Centered Approach

Measure Fluid Intake

Competency Sheet: Unit VIII. LP 1

Name of Student: ____________________________________
Equipment Needed
Measuring Device
I & O Form
Pen and Paper

The Student Completed the Following	Yes	No
1. Obtain a list of the most commonly sed fluid containers in the facility and the amounts they hold		
2. Wash your hands		
3. Identify resident		
4. Explain to the resident what you are doing and ask them to help by writing down what amount and kind of fluids they consume (f able to do so)		
5. Record the amount and type of fluid taken each time that it is offered and consumed on the I & O form		
6. Measure and Record all fluids consumed by the resident during your shift		
a. After meals, snacks		
b. Each time fluids are offered and consumed		
c. Check water pitcher for amount consumed on the shift		
7. Wash hands		
8. Total the amounts at the end of the shift and record in the medical/clinical record		
9. Wash hands.		

The student/employee has satisfactorily completed the procedure and demonstrated competency for the skill: "**Measure Fluid Intake**" according to the steps outlined. Ask the student/employee questions about the procedure to assure they understand the process and what the information is used for.

______________________________________ ____________

Instructor/Clinical Supervisor Signature Date

Measure Fluid Output

Competency Sheet: Unit VIII. LP 1

Name of Student: ______________________________

Equipment Needed

Measuring Device
I & O Form
Gloves

The Student Completed the Following	Yes	No
1. Wash your hands		
2. Put on Gloves		
3. Identify Resident and Explain to the resident what you are doing		
4. Utilize measuring device (graduated container, toilet hat). Put gloves on before handling. Read at eye level.		
5. Measure and record for each time the resident voids and note the number of liquid stools or any emesis on the I & O Form		
6. Remove gloves		
7. Wash hands		
8. Total the amounts at the end of the shift and record in the medical/clinical record		

The student/employee has satisfactorily completed the procedure and demonstrated competency for the skill: "**Measure Fluid Output**" according to the steps outlined. Ask the student/employee questions about the procedure to assure they understand the process and what the information is used for.

______________________________ ____________

Instructor/Clinical Supervisor Signature Date

Becoming a Certified Nurse Assistant: A Person-Centered Approach

Giving Effective & Thorough Report

Competency Sheet: Unit III, LP 2

Name of Student: ________________________________

Equipment Needed:
Assignment Sheet for Shift
Notes that you have taken today

The Student Completed the Following	Yes	No
1. Gathered Shift Assignment Sheet and Notes you have taken.		
2. Identify and greet the charge nurse or the oncoming person accepting your assignment.		
3. Review the assignment list of residents you had today.		
4. Talk about everyone on your list. The kind of day they had, any issues, anything going on, special procedures, incidents/accidents, change in condition, etc. be thorough.		
5. Point out anything that needs follow-up. (Checking VS after a fall or noted change of condition that the next shift will need to incorporate into their shift duties)		
6. Provide opportunity for asking questions and clarifying information.		
7. Be sure you include anything that you'd want to make sure you knew to comfortably start your assignment and keep your residents safe and secure.		

The student/employee has satisfactorily completed the procedure and demonstrated competency for the skill: "**Giving Effective & Thorough Report**" according to the steps outlined. Ask the student/employee questions about the procedure to assure they understand the process and what the information is used for.

________________________________ ________________________________

Instructor/Clinical Supervisor Signature Date

Shave Resident with Disposable Razor

Competency Sheet Unit X, LP 1

Name of Student: ___________________________

Equipment Needed:

Basin/Sink with hot water	Face Towel/washcloth
Disposable Razor	Mirror
Shaving Cream	Aftershave lotion
Gloves	
Towel	

The Student Completed the Following	Yes	No
1. Gather equipment		
2. Identify and greet the resident and introduce yourself		
3. Wash hands- and put-on gloves		
4. Explain what you are going to do		
5. Provide privacy		
6. Position the resident in chair or sitting position in bed in well-lit private area.		
7. Spread towel under resident's chin		
8. Wet face with warm water. If the beard is tough lay the washcloth over the face for a minute or so to soften it. Apply shaving cream 1/8" thick to the face.		
9. Leave lather in place 15-30 seconds.		
10. Hold razor at 45-degree angle to the resident's skin. Start stroking downward with razor under sideburns and work downward over the cheek. Shave in the same direction as the hair grows.		
11. Continue over the chin. Work upward on the neck. Use short, firm strokes. Rinsing the razor often in water.		
12. Shave around lips and under nose carefully. You may have to stretch the skin gently to shave in the creases and sensitive areas or have the resident push their tongue against the crease to expand it to make it easier to shave.		
13. Wash entire face and remove all shave cream.		
14. Pat face dry with towel		

15. Apply after shave (optional).		
16. Clean, store and remove equipment. Dispose of razor in approved sharps container do not recap the razor.		
17. Wash your hands.		
18. Make resident comfortable and assure call light is in reach		
19. Record observations and report anything unusual to charge nurse. If any nicks apply pressure until oozing stops and notify the charge nurse.		

The student/employee has satisfactorily completed the procedure and demonstrated competency for the skill: "**Shave Resident with Disposable Razor"** according to the steps outlined. Ask the student/employee questions about the procedure to assure they understand the process and what the information is used for.

____________________________________ __________

Instructor/Clinical Supervisor Signature Date

Becoming a Certified Nurse Assistant: A Person-Centered Approach

Shave Resident with Electric Razor

Competency Sheet Unit X, LP 1

Name of Student: ______________________________

Equipment Needed:

Basin/Sink with hot water	**Face Towel/washcloth**
Electric Razor	**Mirror**
Pres-shave lotion	**Aftershave lotion**
Gloves	**Towel**

The Student Completed the Following	Yes	No
1. Gather equipment		
2. Identify and greet the resident and introduce yourself		
3. Wash hands- and put-on gloves		
4. Explain what you are going to do		
5. Provide privacy		
6. Position the resident in chair or sitting position in bed in well-lit private area.		
7. Spread towel under resident's chin		
8. Sanitize razor following facility policy.		
9. Leave lather in place 15-30 seconds.		
10. Wash face with soap and water to remove dirt, oil and pat dry		
11. Apply pre-shave lotion if requested		
12. Start shaving from sideburns, holding skintight and using circular motions, shave neck and around mouth.		
13. Apply after shave (optional).		
14. Clean, store and remove equipment. Sanitize razor head using facility policy		
15. Wash your hands.		
16. Make resident comfortable and assure call light is in reach		
17. Record observations and report anything unusual to charge nurse. If any nicks apply pressure until oozing stops and notify the charge nurse.		

The student/employee has satisfactorily completed the procedure and demonstrated competency for the skill: "**Shave Resident with Electric Razor"** according to the steps outlined. Ask the student/employee questions about the procedure to assure they understand the process and what the information is used for.

______________________________ ____________

Instructor/Clinical Supervisor Signature

Becoming a Certified Nurse Assistant: A Person-Centered Approach

Assist with Oral Hygiene

Competency Sheet- Unit VIII, LP 2

Name of Student: ______________________________

Equipment Needed:

Cup or glass	Toothpaste or powder
Emesis basin or sink	Mouthwash
Water	Lip Balm
Toothbrush	Gloves
Hand towel	

The Student Completed the Following	Yes	No
1. Gather equipment		
2. Identify and greet the resident and introduce yourself		
3. Wash hands- and put-on gloves		
4. Explain what you are going to do		
5. Provide privacy		
6. Dilute mouthwash (1 Oz mouthwash 1 Oz water) and assist resident to upright position or bathroom over the sink		
7. Pour water over toothbrush; instructor assist resident to put a small amount of toothpaste on brush		
8. Instructor assist resident to brush along gum line then brush teeth up and down on both sides.		
9. Brush the biting surfaces of the molars (back teeth) with a back-and-forth motion		
10. Gently brush the tongue		
11. Instructors assist the resident to rinse his/her mouth with water, hold emesis basin under resident's chin with one hand. Instruct to spit into basin or sink and wipe lips with towel.		

12. Provide the mouthwash and instruct resident to swish around in mouth and spit out, caution not to swallow. Spit into basin or sink and wipe lips with towel		
13. Lubricate lips with lip balm		
14. Remove, clean and store equipment		
15. Remove gloves and dispose of appropriately		
16. Wash resident's hands and then wash your own.		
17. Make resident comfortable and assure call light is in reach		
18. Record observations and report anything unusual to charge nurse		

The student/employee has satisfactorily completed the procedure and demonstrated competency for the skill: "**Assist with Oral Hygiene"** according to the steps outlined. Ask the student/employee questions about the procedure to assure they understand the process and what the information is used for.

_______________________________________ ___________

Instructor/Clinical Supervisor Signature Date

Becoming a Certified Nurse Assistant: A Person-Centered Approach

Administer Oral Care to Comatose Resident

Competency Sheet Unit VIII, LP

Name of Student: ______________________________

Equipment Needed:

Cup or glass	
Emesis basin or sink	**Mouthwash**
Water	**Lip Balm**
Toothbrush	**Gloves**
Hand towel	

The Student Completed the Following	Yes	No
1. Gather equipment		
2. Identify and greet the resident and introduce yourself		
3. Wash hands- and put-on gloves		
4. Explain what you are going to do		
5. Provide privacy		
6. Dilute mouthwash (1 Oz mouthwash 1 Oz water) . Move resident to the side of the bed nearest you. Turn head to the side.		
7. Spread towel under resident's chin		
8. Moisten washcloth over emesis basin with diluted mouthwash		
9. Clean teeth and gums by wrapping wet washcloth around a tongue depressor or uses a commercial mouthwash swab.		
10. Clean the tongue with the washcloth or swab and inside surfaces of the mouth		
11. Moisten toothbrush with diluted mouthwash brush gumline and teeth in up and down motions on both sides,		
12. Wipe lips with a towel		
13. Lubricate lips with lip balm		
14. Remove, clean and store equipment		
15. Remove gloves and dispose of appropriately		
16. Wash resident's hands and then wash your own.		

17. Make resident comfortable and assure call light is in reach		
18. Record observations and report anything unusual to charge nurse		

The student/employee has satisfactorily completed the procedure and demonstrated competency for the skill: "**Administer Oral Care to Comatose Resident"** according to the steps outlined. Ask the student/employee questions about the procedure to assure they understand the process and what the information is used for.

_______________________________________ __________

Instructor/Clinical Supervisor Signature Date

Becoming a Certified Nurse Assistant: A Person-Centered Approach

Provide Denture Care

Competency Sheet: Unit VIII, LP 2

Name of Student: ____

Equipment Needed:

Cup or glass	Denture Cleanser (Toothpaste)
Emesis basin or sink	Mouthwash
Water	Denture Cup
Toothbrush	Lip Balm
Hand towel	Gloves

The Student Completed the Following	Yes	No
1. Gather equipment		
2. Identify and greet the resident and introduce yourself		
3. Wash hands and put on gloves		
4. Explain what you are going to do		
5. Provide privacy		
6. Ask the resident to remove dentures or run your finger along the top of the upper gum as you gently push the upper edge of the denture forward and down. Lower dentures can be removed by running your gloved finger along the lower gum line; push forward and up		
7. Place denture in clean denture cup marked with resident's name.		
8. Provide water or diluted mouthwash to rinse mouth of food particles. If desired, allow resident or assist resident to brush gums and tongue with soft brush to clean gums and tongue and stimulate circulation.		
9. Allow resident to spit into emesis basis or sink. Inspect the gums and mouth for any sores, irritation, etc.		
10. Provide towel or tissue to wipe resident's mouth or encourage them to do so themselves.		
11. Apply lip balm to resident's lips or allow them to do so themselves.		
12. Fill clean sink with 3-4 inches of cool water. Place a clean washcloth on the bottom of the sink (may help to prevent breakage if you drop them in the sink)		

13. Brush dentures thoroughly using toothbrush and denture cleanser or toothpaste.		
14. Rinse denture with cool running water and place in clean cup.		
15. If resident wants to wear dentures, replace them in the mouth (upper plate first)		
16. If resident is not going to wear dentures, store them in a clean denture cup filled with appropriate solution (facility policy or resident care plan)		
17. Remove, clean and store equipment		
18. Remove gloves and dispose of appropriately		
19. Wash resident's hands and then wash your own.		
20. Make resident comfortable and assure call light is in reach		
21. Record observations and report anything unusual to charge nurse		

The student/employee has satisfactorily completed the procedure and demonstrated competency for the skill: "**Provide Denture Care"** according to the steps outlined. Ask the student/employee questions about the procedure to assure they understand the process and what the information is used for.

____ ____________

Instructor/Clinical Supervisor Signature Date

Provide Fingernail Care

Competency Sheet-Unit X, LP 1

Name of Student: ________________________________

Equipment Needed:

Wash basin ¾ full warm, soapy water	**Pitcher of warm water**
Towel and Paper Towels	**Disposable or reusable bed protector**
Orange Stick	**Emery Board**
Nail Clippers	**Alcohol Swabs**
Lotion	**Gloves/Goggles (if needed)**

The Student Completed the Following	Yes	No
1. Gather equipment		
2. Identify and greet the resident and introduce yourself		
3. Wash hands- and put-on gloves		
4. Explain what you are going to do		
5. Provide privacy		
6. Set resident in chair or position in upright position in bed. Place disposable or reusable bed protector under the hands and place the towel of the protector		
7. Place basin of warm, soapy water on towel/bed protector and place residents' hands in basin.		
8. Soak fingers in the basin for 5-10 minutes		
9. Rinse hands with clear, warm water and dry with towel. Remove basin when finished soaking.		
10. Place towel under residents' hands		
11. Using the orange stick gently remove dirt and debris from around and under each fingernail. Use the paper towel to clean the orange stick.		
12. Put on goggle to trim nails if the are thick and extremely hard. Trim nails as needed. Disinfect the clippers with alcohol swabs before and after using them.		
13. Shape and smooth the nails with the emery board.		
14. Rub lotion into hands providing massage, circular motions.		

15. Remove gloves (if used) and dispose of appropriately		
16. Remove, clean and store equipment. Again, assure clippers are cleaned with alcohol after use.		
17. Wash your hands.		
18. Make resident comfortable and assure call light is in reach		
19. Record observations and report anything unusual to charge nurse		

The student/employee has satisfactorily completed the procedure and demonstrated competency for the skill: "**Provide Fingernail Care"** according to the steps outlined. Ask the student/employee questions about the procedure to assure they understand the process and what the information is used for.

____ ___________

Instructor/Clinical Supervisor Signature Date

Becoming a Certified Nurse Assistant: A Person-Centered Approach

Provide Toenail Care

Competency Sheet-Unit X, LP 1

Name of Student: ____

Equipment Needed:

Wash basin ¾ full warm, soapy water	**Pitcher of warm water**
Towel and Paper Towels	**Disposable or reusable bed protector or bathmat**
Orange Stick	**Emery Board**
Nail Clippers	**Alcohol Swabs**
Lotion	**Gloves/Goggles (if needed)**

The Student Completed the Following	**Yes**	**No**
1. Gather equipment		
2. Identify and greet the resident and introduce yourself		
3. Wash hands and put on gloves		
4. Explain what you are going to do		
5. Provide privacy		
6. Set resident in chair or position in upright position in bed. Place disposable or reusable bed protector under the feet and place the towel over the protector. If setting up put bath at on floor and cover with the towel		
7. Place basin of warm, soapy water on towel/bed protector and place residents' feet in basin.		
8. Soak feet in the basin for 5-10 minutes. Wash feet observing between toes and all of each foot		
9. Rinse feet with clear, warm water and dry with towel. Remove basin when finished soaking.		
10. Place towel under residents' feet		
11. Using the orange stick gently remove dirt and debris from around and under each toenail. Use the paper towel to clean the orange stick.		
12. Put on goggle to trim nails if the are thick and extremely hard. Trim nails as needed. Disinfect the clippers with alcohol swabs before and after using them.		
13. Shape and smooth the nails with the emery board.		
14. Rub lotion into feet providing massage, circular motions.		

15. Remove gloves (if used) and dispose of appropriately		
16. Remove, clean and store equipment. Again, assure clippers are cleaned with alcohol after use.		
17. Wash your hands.		
18. Make resident comfortable and assure call light is in reach		
19. Record observations and report anything unusual to charge nurse		

The student/employee has satisfactorily completed the procedure and demonstrated competency for the skill: "**Provide Toenail Care"** according to the steps outlined. Ask the student/employee questions about the procedure to assure they understand the process and what the information is used for.

______________________________________ ___________

Instructor/Clinical Supervisor Signature Date

Becoming a Certified Nurse Assistant: A Person-Centered Approach

Comb/Brush Hair

Competency Sheet-Unit X, LP 1

Name of Student: ______________________________________

Equipment Needed:

Residents Personal Comb/Brush	Hand mirror if available
Towel	

The Student Completed the Following	Yes	No
1. Gather equipment		
2. Identify and greet the resident and introduce yourself		
3. Wash hands- and put-on gloves		
4. Explain what you are going to do		
5. Provide privacy		
6. Place towel over shoulders if sitting up or over pillow if in bed.		
7. Remove eyeglasses, hairpins, bands, etc. and set aside		
8. Brush or comb hair gently using downward strokes. To remove tangles, start at the bottom of the hair and work toward the scalp.		
9. Arrange hair as resident requests		
10. Allow resident to look in mirror. Replace eyeglasses		
11. Remove, clean and store equipment. Again, assure clippers are cleaned with alcohol after use.		
12. Wash your hands.		
13. Make resident comfortable and assure call light is in reach		
14. Record observations and report anything unusual to charge nurse		

The student/employee has satisfactorily completed the procedure and demonstrated competency for the skill: "**Comb/Brush Hair**" according to the steps outlined. Ask the student/employee questions about the procedure to assure they understand the process and what the information is used for.

______________________________________ ____________

Instructor/Clinical Supervisor Signature Date

Becoming a Certified Nurse Assistant: A Person-Centered Approach

Provide Shampoo During Tub/Shower Bath

Competency Sheet- Unit X, LP 1

Name of Student: ______________________________

Equipment Needed:

Bath Towel (2)	**Face Towel/washcloth**
Shampoo	**Cream Rinse (optional)**
Bath Thermometer	**Pitcher/handheld shower nozzle**
Hair Dryer (resident room use)	**Resident's personal brush/comb**
Hand mirror if available	**Curlers/Rollers (optional)**

The Student Completed the Following	Yes	No
1. Gather equipment		
2. Identify and greet the resident and introduce yourself		
3. Wash hands- and put-on gloves		
4. Explain what you are going to do		
5. Provide privacy		
6. Adjust water temp to 105 degrees F. Position resident in tub or shower appropriately		
7. Ask resident to hold folded washcloth/face towel over eyes		
8. Apply water to hair until it is completely wet (nozzle or pitcher)		
9. Apply small amount of shampoo, lather massaging well with fingers. Inspect scalp while shampooing and rinsing		
10. Rinse thoroughly, working from front to back		
11. Repeat steps 9 and 10 if necessary		
12. Use cream rinse or vinegar rinse (optional) and rinse hair again.		
13. Towel dry hair		
14. Encourage resident to comb or brush hair, apply rollers (optional)		
15. Dry hair quickly, remove curlers when hair is dried if used.		
16. Let resident use mirror and make comfortable		

17. Wash your hands.		
18. Make resident comfortable and assure call light is in reach		
19. Record observations and report anything unusual to charge nurse		

The student/employee has satisfactorily completed the procedure and demonstrated competency for the skill: "**Provide Shampoo During Tub/Shower Bath"** according to the steps outlined. Ask the student/employee questions about the procedure to assure they understand the process and what the information is used for.

____ ___________

Instructor/Clinical Supervisor Signature Date

Provide Bed Shampoo

Competency Sheet- Unit X, LP 1

Name of Student: ____

Equipment Needed:

Bath Towel (2)	**Face Towel/washcloth**
Shampoo & Cream Rinse (optional)	**Bath Blanket**
Cotton Balls	**Basin or pitcher with warm water**
Hair Dryer (resident room use)	**Resident's personal brush/comb**
Hand Mirror and Curlers/Rollers (optional)	**Second basin or bucket for draining water and footstool or chair to place bucket in**
Waterproof bed protector	**Shampoo Trough**

The Student Completed the Following	**Yes**	**No**
1. Gather equipment		
2. Identify and greet the resident and introduce yourself		
3. Wash hands- and put-on gloves		
4. Explain what you are going to do		
5. Provide privacy		
6. Raise the bed to the highest position		
7. Place empty bucket on chair or footstool with the end of the shampoo trough in it to drain the water into the bucket		
8. Remove the pillow. Place a towel under the head and across the shoulders.		
9. Move resident to the side of the bed and place the shampoo trough under the head on top of the waterproof bed protector, with end extended to the empty bucket. Cover with bath blanket and fanfold top sheet and blanket to foot of bed. Place cotton balls in resident's ears. Ask resident to hold folded washcloth/face towel over eyes		
10. Apply water to hair until it is completely wet (pitcher)		
11. Apply small amount of shampoo, lather massaging well with fingers. Inspect scalp while shampooing and rinsing		
12. Rinse thoroughly, working from front to back		

13. Repeat steps 9 and 10 if necessary		
14. Use cream rinse or vinegar rinse (optional) and rinse hair again.		
15. Towel dry hair. Remove cotton balls from ears.		
16. Encourage resident to comb or brush hair, apply rollers (optional)		
17. Clean, store and remove equipment.		
18. Dry hair quickly, remove curlers when hair is dried if used		
19. Let resident use mirror and make comfortable		
20. Wash your hands. Return bed to lower position		
21. Make resident comfortable and assure call light is in reach		
22. Record observations and report anything unusual to charge nurse		

The student/employee has satisfactorily completed the procedure and demonstrated competency for the skill: "**Provide Bed Shampoo"** according to the steps outlined. Ask the student/employee questions about the procedure to assure they understand the process and what the information is used for.

____ __________

Instructor/Clinical Supervisor Signature Date

Becoming a Certified Nurse Assistant: A Person-Centered Approach

Give Peri Care with Catheter

Competency Sheet-Unit IX, LP 1

Name of Student: ________________________________

Equipment Needed:

Basin of warm water	Bath Blanket
Washcloths 3-4	Gloves
Mild soap	
Disposable or reusable bed protector	
Towel	

The Student Completed the Following	Yes	No
1. Gather equipment		
2. Identify and greet the resident and introduce yourself		
3. Wash hands and put on gloves		
4. Explain what you are going to do		
5. Provide privacy		
6. Resident should be in supine position with legs apart; place bed protector under buttocks		
7. Cover with bath blanket then remove top sheet		
8. Check catheter and drainage bag for leaks, kinks, level of bag, color and clarity of urine; ensure drainage bag is securely attached to bed frame.		
9. Expose the perineal area. Female: Separate labia and gently wash around the opening of the urethra with soap and water. Male: uncircumcised, gently pull back foreskin and wash around the opening of the urethra with soap and water, if circumcised wash around opening of urethra with soap and water.		
10. Wash catheter tubing from the opening of the urethra outward 4 inches or farther as needed. Do not pull on the catheter		
11. With a fresh washcloth wash one side of the labia on the female and use a clean area of the washcloth to wash the other side. Wiping from front to back Males wash tip of penis down toward the scrotum.		
12. Turn resident to side and wash annual folds and anus with a fresh washcloth moving from the bottom up toward the coccyx.		

13. Inspect the skin front and back looking for irritation sores or anything unusual. Inspect catheter entrance around urethra noting any blood or other discharge		
14. Remove bed protector and bath blanket. Place soiled linens in dirty linen container.		
15. Remove, clean and store equipment		
16. Remove gloves and dispose of appropriately		
17. Wash resident's hands and then wash your own.		
18. Make resident comfortable and assure call light is in reach		
19. Record observations and report anything unusual to charge nurse		

The student/employee has satisfactorily completed the procedure and demonstrated competency for the skill: "**Giver Peri Care with A Catheter"** according to the steps outlined. Ask the student/employee questions about the procedure to assure they understand the process and what the information is used for.

_______________________________________ ___________

Instructor/Clinical Supervisor Signature Date

Becoming a Certified Nurse Assistant: A Person-Centered Approach

Assist Resident in Using Bedpan

Competency Sheet-Unit IX, LP 1

Name of Student: ___________________________________

Equipment Needed:

Bedpan and Cover	
Gloves	
Toilet Paper	

The Student Completed the Following	**Yes**	**No**
1. Gather equipment		
2. Identify and greet the resident and introduce yourself		
3. Wash hands- and put-on gloves		
4. Explain what you are going to do		
5. Provide privacy		
6. Resident should be in supine position lying on back turn back top bedding. (May sprinkle powder on bedpan to prevent sticking)		
Resident is Able to Help		
7. Have resident flex knees and lift buttocks off mattress		
8. Slip bedpan under the resident's hips and adjust		
Resident Unable to Help		
9. Turn resident on side facing away from you		
10. Expose buttocks and position bedpan firmly against buttocks		
11. Place small pillow or rolled towel at top of bedpan at the small of the resident's back		
12. Turn resident toward you and onto the bedpan		
13. Raise the head of bed, if allowed, assure privacy and call light in reach and toilet tissue		
14. Remove gloves, wash hands and leave the room		

15. Return to room promptly when resident calls on call light or check on them after 5 minutes (DO NOT Leave a resident on a bedpan for more than 10 minutes. This can lead to discomfort and skin breakdown		
16. If resident can assist place on hand under the small of the back and assist the resident to lift his/her hips while you pull the bedpan out with the other hand. If unable to assist, hold bedpan with one hand and roll resident off pan with other hand. This should prevent contents from spilling		
17. Remove pan and cover it. Wipe, wash and dry the perineal area from front to back.		
18. Take pan to bathroom, note color and clarity of urine, measure and record I & O if applicable and empty into the toilet.		
19. Remove, clean and store equipment		
20. Remove gloves and dispose of appropriately		
21. Wash resident's hands and then wash your own.		
22. Make resident comfortable and assure call light is in reach		
23. Record observations and report anything unusual to charge nurse		

The student/employee has satisfactorily completed the procedure and demonstrated competency for the skill: "**Assist Resident in Using Bedpan"** according to the steps outlined. Ask the student/employee questions about the procedure to assure they understand the process and what the information is used for.

____________________________________ __________

Instructor/Clinical Supervisor Signature Date

Becoming a Certified Nurse Assistant: A Person-Centered Approach

Assist Resident in Using Urinal

Competency Sheet-Unit IX, LP 1

Name of Student: ______________________________

Equipment Needed:

Urinal and Cover	
Gloves	
Toilet Paper	

The Student Completed the Following	Yes	No
1. Gather equipment		
2. Identify and greet the resident and introduce yourself		
3. Wash hands- and put-on gloves		
4. Explain what you are going to do		
5. Provide privacy		
6. Turn back top bedding, except for top sheet. Expose peri area. Place the resident's penis in the urinal and lay the urinal between the legs. Make sure there is no pressure on the scrotum.		
7. Make sure urinal is at an angle to keep from spilling out. Flat edge should be lying on the bed.		
8. Remove gloves, wash hands, and leave the room		
9. Return to room promptly when resident calls on call light or check on them after 5 minutes (DO NOT Leave a urinal in place for more than 10 minutes. This can lead to discomfort and skin breakdown Wash hands- and put-on gloves.		
10. Remove urinal and cover it.		
11. Take urinal to bathroom, note color and clarity of urine, measure and record I & O if applicable and empty into the toilet.		
12. Remove, clean and store equipment		
13. Remove gloves and dispose of appropriately		
14. Wash resident's hands and then wash your own.		
15. Make resident comfortable and assure call light is in reach		
16. Record observations and report anything unusual to charge nurse		

The student/employee has satisfactorily completed the procedure and demonstrated competency for the skill: "**Assist Resident in Using Urinal"** according to the steps outlined. Ask the student/employee questions about the procedure to assure they understand the process and what the information is used for.

______________________________________ ____________

Instructor/Clinical Supervisor Signature Date

Becoming a Certified Nurse Assistant: A Person-Centered Approach

Change Urinary Drainage Bag

Competency Sheet-Unit IX, LP 1

Name of Student: ____

Equipment Needed:

New Urinary Drainage Bag or Leg Bag	Alcohol Swabs 2
Gloves	

The Student Completed the Following	Yes	No
1. Gather equipment		
2. Identify and greet the resident and introduce yourself		
3. Wash hands- and put-on gloves		
4. Explain what you are going to do		
5. Provide privacy		
6. Crimp with your fingers or close clamp on tubing so urine does not flow.		
7. Disconnect catheter tubing from drainage bag and swab end of catheter tubing with alcohol. Connect the new bag to the tubing.		
8. Unclamp tubing so urine can flow again. Follow facility policy regarding marking date and time on new drainage bag of the change.		
9. Assure leg bag is strapped or drainage bag is securely fastened to unmovable surface such as bed frame)		
10. Remove, clean and store equipment		
11. Remove gloves and dispose of appropriately		
12. Wash resident's hands and then wash your own.		
13. Make resident comfortable and assure call light is in reach		
14. Record observations and report anything unusual to charge nurse		

The student/employee has satisfactorily completed the procedure and demonstrated competency for the skill: "**Change Urinary Drainage Bag"** according to the steps outlined. Ask the student/employee questions about the procedure to assure they understand the process and what the information is used for.

____ ____________

Instructor/Clinical Supervisor Signature Date

Becoming a Certified Nurse Assistant: A Person-Centered Approach

Empty Urinary Drainage Bag

Competency Sheet-Unit IX, LP 1

Name of Student: ______________________________________

Equipment Needed:

Graduate or Measuring Device	
Gloves	
Alcohol Swabs 2	

The Student Completed the Following	Yes	No
1. Gather equipment		
2. Identify and greet the resident and introduce yourself		
3. Wash hands- and put-on gloves		
4. Explain what you are going to do		
5. Provide privacy		
6. Place graduate under the drain at the bottom of the bag.		
7. Open drain and allow urine to empty into measuring device. Being careful not to allow the drain tube to touch the inside of the measuring device. If it does wipe the drain with alcohol swabs to disinfect.		
8. Close the drain with the clamp and replace it in the holder of the bag.		
9. Note, color, clarity and amount, record on I & O Sheet, empty urine into the toilet and flush.		
10. Remove, clean and store equipment		
11. Remove gloves and dispose of appropriately		
12. Wash resident's hands and then wash your own.		
13. Make resident comfortable and assure call light is in reach		
14. Record observations and report anything unusual to charge nurse		

The student/employee has satisfactorily completed the procedure and demonstrated competency for the skill: "**Empty Urinary Drainage Bag"** according to the steps outlined. Ask the student/employee questions about the procedure to assure they understand the process and what the information is used for.

______________________________________ ____________

Instructor/Clinical Supervisor Signature Date

Becoming a Certified Nurse Assistant: A Person-Centered Approach

Collecting a Urine or a Clean-Catch Urine Sample

Competency Sheet: Unit VII. LP 2

Name of Student: ______________________________

Equipment Needed:

Bedpan, urinal, or toilet hat
Specimen container
Labels for Container
At least two pair of gloves
Disposable trash bag
Cleaning solution (if needed)

Remember if you contaminate your gloves during the procedure, remove the contaminated pair, wash hands and re-glove.

The Student Completed the Following	Yes	No
1. Wash and Dry Hands		
2. Assist resident to bedpan, toilet with hat or commode or urinal.		
3. Put on gloves		
4. Pour about 60 cc of urine into the specimen container. Discard the remained by emptying into the toilet.		
5. Close the container securely, write the resident's name, room number, date and time you collected the sample on the container label.		
6. Place the specimen container in a biohazard bag and make sure the bag is properly sealed.		
7. Remove gloves and wash your hands.		
Clean catch Urine Specimen		
8. Wash and Dry Hands		
9. Assist resident to bedpan, toilet with hat or commode or urinal.		
10. Put on gloves		
11. Clean the ureteral opening. For a female, use one wipe to clean one side of the labia and a second wipe to clean the other side, use a third wipe to clean down the middle. Always clean with a single stroke going front to back. Use each wipe only once and discard. For a male, clean the penis following the procedure used for perineal care. Remember to pull back the foreskin for an uncircumcised male,		
12. Have the resident begin to urinate and then stop if they can, Do not collect the first urine. (If they cannot stop the stream of urine you must place the container under the stream before they finish to collect the sample.		
13. Hold the specimen container under the urethra, if they were able to stop, and ask them to begin again to collect the specimen.		
14. Close the container securely, write the resident's name, room number, date and time you collected the sample on the container label.		

15. Place the specimen container in a biohazard bag and make sure the bag is properly sealed.		
16. Remove gloves and wash your hands.		

The student/employee has satisfactorily completed the procedure and demonstrated competency for the skill: "**Collecting a Urine or a Clean-Catch Urine Sample"** according to the steps outlined. Ask the student/employee questions about the procedure to assure they understand the process and what the information is used for.

_______________________________________ ___________

Instructor/Clinical Supervisor Signature Date

Becoming a Certified Nurse Assistant: A Person-Centered Approach

Colostomy Care/ Change Ostomy Pouch (Established/Uncomplicated Colostomy)

Competency Sheet: Unit VII. LP 2

Name of Student: ____

Equipment Needed:

Bath Blanket	Washcloth and Towel
Pouch	Soap and Water
Skin Barrier if ordered	
Measuring Guide	
Plastic Bag	

The Student Completed the Following	Yes	No
1. Gather equipment		
2. Identify and greet the resident and introduce yourself		
3. Wash hands and put on gloves		
4. Explain what you are going to do		
5. Provide privacy		
6. Raise bed to high position. Place bath blanket over resident and fold top lines down to hips		
7. Remove old pouch by pushing against skin as you pull off the pouch. Discard in plastic bag, saving the clip. Note the amount and type of drainage and feces.		
8. Cleanse area around stoma with warm water and soap. Clean the skin of the stoma and rinse with gentle strokes. Pat dry.		
9. Observe stoma and skin surrounding for redness or irritation or breakdown.		
10. Measure stoma with measuring guide. Cut Pouch 1/8 inch larger than measurement to prevent pressure to stoma.		
11. Apply skin barrier paste to peristomal area. Wet gloved fingers and spread paste around stoma.		
12. Remove paper from adhesive area on pouch. Center and apply clean pouch over stoma.		
13. Press adhesive around stoma to form wrinkle free seal. Secure end of pouch with clip if needed some do not have clips.		
14. Remove, clean and store equipment		

15. Remove gloves and dispose of appropriately		
16. Wash resident's hands and then wash your own.		
17. Make resident comfortable and assure call light is in reach		
18. Record observations and report anything unusual to charge nurse		

The student/employee has satisfactorily completed the procedure and demonstrated competency for the skill: "**Colostomy Care and Change Ostomy Bag" (Established/Uncomplicated Colostomy)** according to the steps outlined. Ask the student/employee questions about the procedure to assure they understand the process and what the information is used for.

____________________________________ ____________

Instructor/Clinical Supervisor Signature Date

Becoming a Certified Nurse Assistant: A Person-Centered Approach

Make an Occupied Bed

Competency Sheet-Unit X, LP 1

Name of Student: ______________________________

Equipment Needed:

Pillowcase	**Plastic Pillow Cover (if used)**
Bedspread	**Blanket**
Top Sheet	**Disposable or reusable pad (if used)**
Cotton lift sheet (draw sheet) if used	**Bottom Sheet (Flat or fitted)**
Mattress Pad or cover	**Soiled Linen Bag**
Gloves (optional-if no possible contact with body fluids)	

The Student Completed the Following	Yes	No
1. Gather equipment		
2. Identify and greet the resident and introduce yourself		
3. Wash hands and put on gloves		
4. Explain what you are going to do. Provide privacy.		
5. Raise bed to highest level. Bed should be in flat position if resident can tolerate it. If the bed has a side rail or partial rail put it up on the side, you are not working on.		
6. Loosen the top of the bedding at foot of bed.		
7. Remove spread, fold spread to foot of bed. Remove by grasping center and place on back of chair.		
8. Remove blanket according to above procedure.		
9. Place bath blanket over top sheet. Ask resident to hold blanket in place or tuck under resident's shoulders. Remove top sheet and place in linen container.		
10. Keep pillow under resident's head and turn resident to side of bed you are not making.		
11. Loosen bottom bedding; free bottom linen and roll each piece to the resident's back.		
12. Remove gloves and dispose, wash hands. Make sure bed rails are up if available or lower bed while you step away.		

13. Place mattress pad on bed lengthwise with fold in center.		
14. Place bottom sheet lengthwise with fold in center and lower edge of sheet even with foot of mattress.		
15. Tuck sheet under head of mattress if flat sheet miter corners tuck well under the mattress.		
16. Fanfold bottom sheet close to resident's back.		
17. Center lift sheet if used and incontinence pad over that and fan fold to resident's back. Tuck lift sheet in under the mattress.		
18. Raise that bed rail, assist the resident to turn facing you and moving to the clean side of the bed. Walk around to the other side of the bed.		
19. Move and keep pillow under resident's head.		
20. Pull through all bottom linen and tuck appropriately and assure all wrinkles are out of linen, remove and discard soiled linen and place in linen bag. Keep used linen off the floor, bedside table and away from your uniform.		
21. Pull the sheet toward the bottom of the bed and tuck under mattress (miter corners if a flat sheet)		
22. Assist resident to center of bed.		
23. Place top sheet over bath blanket and then remove bath blanket and place in soiled linen.		
24. If blanket and bedspread are used add to the top sheet.		
25. Change pillowcase and place under resident's head.		
26. Lower bed rails if used and not ordered by the physician and return bed to lower position. Assure crank is tucked in.		
27. Make resident comfortable and assure call light is within reach. .		
28. Wash your hands		

The student/employee has satisfactorily completed the procedure and demonstrated competency for the skill: "**Make an Occupied Bed"** according to the steps outlined. Ask the student/employee questions about the procedure to assure they understand the process and what the information is used for.

____________________________________ __________

Instructor/Clinical Supervisor Signature Date

Make an Unoccupied Bed

Name of Student: ____

Equipment Needed:

Pillowcase	**Plastic Pillow Cover (if used)**
Bedspread	**Blanket**
Top Sheet	**Disposable or reusable pad (if used)**
Cotton lift sheet (draw sheet) if used	**Bottom Sheet (Flat or fitted)**
Mattress Pad or cover	**Soiled Linen Bag**
Gloves (optional-if no possible contact with body fluids)	

The Student Completed the Following	Yes	No
1. Gather equipment		
2. Identify and greet the resident and introduce yourself		
3. Wash hands- and put-on gloves		
4. Explain what you are going to do		
5. Raise bed to highest level. Bed should be in flat position.		
6. Remove pillow and strip pillowcase.		
7. Strip bed and place soiled linen in soiled linen bag. Do not place on floor, do not fan or fold, do not let them touch your uniform.		
8. Wash and dry mattress if soiled-follow facility policy		
9. Remove gloves if warn and dispose of. Wash hands		
10. If used, place mattress pad on bed and pull smooth.		
11. Unfold bottom sheet on bed, full length, with bottom hem at bottom edge of mattress. If using fitted sheet, tuck in all four corners securely under the mattress corners		

12. Tuck in head end of bottom sheet if not a fitted sheet and miter corner.		
13. Tuck in near edge of bottom sheet, working from head to foot.		
14. Fold lift sheet (if used and place over bottom sheet. Add incontinence pad if used)		
15. Place top sheet, halved, full length of bed, with hem at edge of head end of mattress.		
16. Unfold the top sheet and place it level with the top edge of the edge of the head of the mattress.		
17. Place blanket over top sheet centered on bed and about 9 inches down from the edge of the top sheet.		
18. Place bedspread (centered) over top sheet and blanket, leave enough spread to cover pillow at top edge		
19. Miter lower corner of sheet, blanket and spread together on the near side, allow to hang free.		
20. Gather open end of pillowcase in one hand, full length, ad grasp pillow edge with same hand. With free hand, fit pillow corners into case.		
21. Place pillow on near half of bed with open end of case away from the doorway; walk to far side of bed.		
22. Fold back on bed each piece of linen		
23. Pull mattress pad smooth and tuck under mattress from head to foot.		
24. Pull bottom sheet tight; tuck under head of mattress; miter corner; tuck in remainder of sheet from head to foot.		
25. Tighten lift sheet; tuck in middle first, then top 1/3 and finally bottom 1/3.		
26. Pull top sheet, blanket, and bedspread straight, tuck under foot end of mattress.		
27. Miter corner with sheet, blanket, adm spread.		
28. Place pillow in center of head of bed; pull bedspread over.		
29. Lower bed and put bed crank in.		
30. Make resident comfortable and assure call light is within reach. .		
31. Wash your hands		

The student/employee has satisfactorily completed the procedure and demonstrated competency for the skill: "**Make an Unoccupied Bed"** according to the steps outlined. Ask the student/employee questions about the procedure to assure they understand the process and what the information is used for.

______________________________________ __________

Instructor/Clinical Supervisor Signature Date

Complete Shower Bath

Name of Student: ____

Equipment Needed:

Bath Thermometer	**Soap**
Bath Towels (3-4)	**Face Towel**
Washcloths (3-4)	**Bath Blanket**
Lotion	**Deodorant**
Powder (optional)	**Linen Bag**
Clean Cloths	**Gown or Pajamas**
Shower chair	**Shower cap (optional)**
Equipment for Hair Care	**Bath Floor Mat**
Resident's Toiletries, makeup	**Gloves**
Disinfectant solution and cleaning cloth	**Nonskid bathmat or towel**

The Student Completed the Following	Yes	No
1. Gather equipment		
2. Identify and greet the resident and introduce yourself		
3. Wash hands- and put-on gloves		
4. Explain what you are going to do		
5. Provide privacy		
6. See that the Shower room is free of drafts and between the temperature of 75-80 degrees F.		
7. Ensure the shower chair are clean. Disinfect per facility's policy		
8. Place nonskid mat in shower stall if resident will be standing at all.		
9. Bring resident to shower room or if brought to you greet resident introduce yourself and explain what you are going to do.		

10. Wash your hands- and put-on gloves		
11. Offering toileting.		
12. If resident is dressed undress a put-on robe and slippers		
13. Ambulate or transport to tub room or assist resident to the shower chair.		
14. Fill tub with warm water 105 degrees F use bath thermometer or test with your inside of wrist.		
15. Assist to remove robe and slippers or undress if/she has not already done so.		
16. Assist resident into shower chair. Adjust shower spray to 95-105 degrees F. Direct spray away from resident while adjusting. Check water on inside of wrist if bath thermometer is not available.		
17. Assist resident as needed in washing. If resident is unable to help, start with eyes, then wash face, ears, neck, arms, hands, chest, abdomen and back.		
18. Rinse with warm water		
19. Wash, rinse and dry the neck		
20. Wash legs, feet, and between toes. Rinse well with warm water; discard washcloth in linen container.		
21. A shampoo can be given at this time. Cover hair with towel after completing		
22. Wash peri-area from front to back. Wash female labia from front of chair, anal area from under chair.		
23. Wash between buttocks and discard washcloth in soiled laundry container. Rinse well from front to back.		
24. Assist resident out of shower, cover with bath blanket		
25. Remove and discard gloves. Wash hands.		
26. Uncover resident, one area at a time, and pat dry with a towel. Once towel has been used below the waist put in soiled linen and do not use again on area above the waist.		
27. Apply powder, lotion, and deodorant if desired.		
28. Assist with dressing		
29. Return to resident room and provide personal care such as shaving, nail care and hair care.		
30. Make resident comfortable and assure call light is within reach. .		
31. Return to shower room disinfect shower chair per facility policy		
32. Clean, store equipment		
33. Wash your hands		

34. Record observations and report anything unusual to the charge nurse.		

The student/employee has satisfactorily completed the procedure and demonstrated competency for the skill: "**Complete Shower Bath"** according to the steps outlined. Ask the student/employee questions about the procedure to assure they understand the process and what the information is used for.

_______________________________________ ____________

Instructor/Clinical Supervisor Signature Date

Complete Bed Bath

Name of Student: ______________________________________

Equipment Needed:

Bath Basin	**Soap and Soap Dish**
Bath Towels (3-4)	**Face Towel**
Washcloths (3-4)	**Bath Blanket**
Lotion	**Deodorant**
Powder (optional)	**Linen Bag**
Clean Bed Linen	**Gown or Pajamas**
Equipment for Oral Hygiene	**Equipment for Shaving**
Equipment for Hair Care	**Equipment for Nail Care**
Resident's Toiletries, makeup	**Gloves**
Bedpan/Urinal	

The Student Completed the Following	**Yes**	**No**
1. Gather equipment		
2. Identify and greet the resident and introduce yourself		
3. Wash hands- and put-on gloves		
4. Explain what you are going to do		
5. Provide privacy		
6. Assist with oral hygiene and shaving if applicable		
7. Offer bedpan/urinal then empty, clean, and put away		
8. Remove gloves and discard. Wash hands- and put-on clean gloves		
9. Place resident in supine position near the side of the bed nearest you. Raise the bed to a comfortable level.		
10. Untuck bed linens		

11. Remove bedspread and blanket; fold and place on chair if reusing otherwise place in soiled linen bag		
12. Cover top sheet with bath blanket and ask resident to hold bath blanket in place, if unable tuck under the shoulders and remove the top sheet and place in soiled linen bag.		
13. Remove resident's gown or pajamas and place in soiled linen bag.		
14. Fill bath basin 2/3 warm water (115 degrees F) Check temperature with bath thermometer or inside of wrist.		
15. Place towel across resident's chest		
16. Wet washcloth, squeeze out excess water and make a washcloth mitt.		
17. Wash eyes first. Start at inner corner and work out. Use a different area of the washcloth for the other eye. Don't dangle the washcloth ends and DO NOT USE SOAP ON THE EYES		
18. Place towel across chest and fold the bath blanket to the waist.		
19. Wash, rinse and dry chests and breasts while lifting the towel so as not to expose the resident unnecessarily.		
20. Wash, rinse and dry face, ears, nose and mouth. Ask about preference for soap being used on the face.		
21. Wash, rinse and dry the neck		
22. Expose arm farthest from you, place bath towel under arm up to axilla.		
23. Place basin on bed and place resident's hand in basin to soak nails and wash hand.		
24. Wash and rinse far shoulder, axilla, arm and hand.		
25. Remove the basin and dry that side of upper body that you just washed.		
26. Repeat steps 22 through 25 with arm nearest you.		
27. Perform nail care at this time.		
28. Fold blanket to pubic area. Keep chest covered with towel.		
29. Wash, rinse, and dry abdomen. Remove towel and cover with a bath blanket.		
30. Change water in bath basin. Obtain clean washcloth		
31. Expose the farthest leg; flex (bend) leg and place bath towel lengthwise under the leg up to the buttocks.		
32. May place the resident's foot in bath basin while washing the leg if they can flex their knee to do so to allow nails to soak. Wash foot while it is in basin after washing the leg.		
33. Dry leg, foot and carefully between toes.		
34. Repeat steps 31 through 33 with the leg nearest you. Cover resident with a bath blanket on the areas that you are not working with.		

35. May perform toenail care at this time.		
36. Place towel and washcloth in soiled linen bag and get clean ones.		
37. Change water in basin. Ask resident to turn on his/her side with back toward you.		
38. Fold bath blanket over resident's side to expose back and buttocks; place a clean towel parallel to resident's back.		
39. Wash, rinse, and dry back and buttocks.		
40. Remove gloves and dispose of. Wash hands		
41. Give backrub using lotion paying special attention to bony prominences		
42. Put on gloves		
43. Turn resident on back; place clean towel under buttocks.		
44. If resident can assist hand him/her a washcloth with soap and instruct to wash and dry the peri area		
45. If unable perform peri care from front to back. Use a clean washcloth for front and back.		
46. Place dirty linen in appropriate container. Remove gloves and wash hands		
47. If resident did own peri-care provide fresh water to wash hands.		
48. Put clean clothing on, comb hair, apply cosmetics if needed.		
49. Clean, store equipment and assure resident's comfort and assure call light is in reach.		
50. Wash your hands		
51. Record observations and report anything unusual to the charge nurse.		

The student/employee has satisfactorily completed the procedure and demonstrated competency for the skill: "**Complete Bed Bath**" according to the steps outlined. Ask the student/employee questions about the procedure to assure they understand the process and what the information is used for.

____________________________________ __________

Instructor/Clinical Supervisor Signature Date

Becoming a Certified Nurse Assistant: A Person-Centered Approach

Give a Backrub

Competency Sheet-Unit X, LP 1

Name of Student: ______________________________

Equipment Needed:

Lotion	**Bath towel (if giving bed bath)**
Washcloth (if giving bed bath)	**Basin with water (if giving bed bath)**
Soap and Soap Dish (if giving bed bath)	**Gloves if needed**

The Student Completed the Following	**Yes**	**No**
1. Gather equipment		
2. Identify and greet the resident and introduce yourself		
3. Wash hands- and put-on gloves if risk for contamination with body fluids.		
4. Explain what you are going to do. Provide privacy.		
5. Position resident on side of bed closest to you then turn resident on his/her side or assist to prone position.		
6. Place bath towel lengthwise, close to resident's back to protect bedding.		
7. Wash, rinse, and dry back (if giving a bed bath or if the back is soiled)		
8. Warm lotion and then apply to entire back. Begin at lower back and apply to both sides of spinal column to neck, across shoulders, and down to lower back. Pay special attention to bony prominences and note any observations of redness, rashes, bruises, etc.		
9. Adjust bed covers and assist resident to a comfortable position.		
10. Place call signal within reach.		
11. Remove gloves and dispose, wash hands.		
12. Clean and store equipment.		
13. Wash your hands and report any observations to charge nurse		

The student/employee has satisfactorily completed the procedure and demonstrated competency for the skill: "**Give Backrub"** according to the steps outlined. Ask the student/employee questions about the procedure to assure they understand the process and what the information is used for.

______________________________ ____________

Instructor/Clinical Supervisor Signature Date

Becoming a Certified Nurse Assistant: A Person-Centered Approach

Provide Stage I Pressure Ulcer Care

Competency Sheet- Unit X, LP 2

Name of Student: ______________________________

Equipment Needed:

Lotion	Bath towel
Washcloth	Basin with water
Soap and Soap Dish (if giving bed bath)	Gloves if needed

The Student Completed the Following	Yes	No
1. Gather equipment		
2. Identify and greet the resident and introduce yourself		
3. Wash hands and put on gloves if risk for contamination with body fluids.		
4. Explain what you are going to do. Provide privacy.		
5. Check Turning Schedule, see care plan and other communication tools.		
6. Observe skin for any reddened areas		
7. Wash, rinse skin area very gently with soap and water if soiled		
8. Provide clean linen as necessary be sure all winkles are out of linens. Check all other bony prominences for any new or emerging reddened areas and assure that no areas exist for additional pressure (lying on catheter tubing, etc.)		
9. Position resident per turning schedule		
10. Place call signal within reach.		
11. Remove gloves and dispose, wash hands.		
12. Clean and store equipment.		
13. Wash your hands, record, and report any observations to charge nurse		

The student/employee has satisfactorily completed the procedure and demonstrated competency for the skill: "**Provide Stage I Pressure Ulcer Care"** according to the steps outlined. Ask the student/employee questions about the procedure to assure they understand the process and what the information is used for.

______________________________ ____________

Instructor/Clinical Supervisor Signature Date

Apply Elastic Stockings (TED Hose)

Name of Student: ____

Equipment Needed:

Elastic Stockings	Assistive Devices Per Care Plan

The Student Completed the Following	Yes	No
1. Gather equipment		
2. Identify and greet the resident and introduce yourself		
3. Wash hands- and put-on gloves		
4. Explain what you are going to do		
5. Provide privacy		
6. Provide Assistive Devices per Care Plan		
7. With resident lying down expose one leg at a time.		
a. Grasp stocking at top with both hands and fold toward toe end with raised seam (if applicable) on the outside		
b. Adjust over resident's toes with opening at the base of toes.		
c. Apply stocking by folding upward toward the body		
d. Check to see that the stocking is applied evenly and smoothly, without wrinkles.		
8. Repeat for the other leg.		
9. Wash your hands		
10. Record observations and report anything unusual to the charge nurse. 11. To remove gently slide the stocking down the legs, over the heel and then remove. See the care plan on instructions for when to remove and cleaning.		

The student/employee has satisfactorily completed the procedure and demonstrated competency for the skill: "**Apply Elastic Stockings (TED Hose)"** according to the steps outlined. Ask the student/employee questions about the procedure to assure they understand the process and what the information is used for.

____ ____________

Instructor/Clinical Supervisor Signature Date

Becoming a Certified Nurse Assistant: A Person-Centered Approach

Ambulate with Gait Belt

Competency Sheet-Unit XI, LP 1

Name of Student: ____

Equipment Needed:

Gait Belt	Chair

The Student Completed the Following	Yes	No
1. Gather equipment		
2. Identify and greet the resident and introduce yourself		
3. Wash hands		
4. Explain what you are going to do		
5. Provide privacy		
6. Provide Assistive Devices per Care Plan		
7. Adjust bed height to low position. Lock brakes on the bed.		
8. Assist resident to the side of the bed and allow time to gain balance. Put on socks and nonskid shoes.		
9. Put on gait belt around resident's waist. Assist to stand using good body mechanics.		
10. Assist resident to stand by straightening legs as you lift with gait belt as resident pushes down with hands on the mattress.		
11. Walk with the resident by placing one hand on gait belt in front of resident's waist and your other hand in back under the gait belt. Walk on the weaker side and encourage resident to use handrail with strong side.		
12. Walk in the same pattern as the resident (both stepping with the left foot at the same time). Assist resident to step forward with the strong foot first.		
13. Ambulate the resident the distance outlined by the charge nurse or plan of care. Remember if the resident loses		

weight-bearing ability use the emergency procedure for assisting with a fall and don't move the resident until assessed by the charge nurse.		
14. Return resident to bed or chair.		
15. Make the resident comfortable, place signal light within reach, Store lift properly.		
16. Wash hands.		

The student/employee has satisfactorily completed the procedure and demonstrated competency for the skill: "**Ambulate with Gait Belt**" according to the steps outlined. Ask the student/employee questions about the procedure to assure they understand the process and what the information is used for.

_______________________________________ ___________

Instructor/Clinical Supervisor Signature Date

Ambulate with Cane

Competency Sheet-Unit XI, LP 1

Name of Student: ______________________________________
Equipment Needed:

Gait Belt	
Cane	

The Student Completed the Following	Yes	No
1. Gather equipment		
2. Identify and greet the resident and introduce yourself		
3. Wash hands		
4. Explain what you are going to do		
5. Provide privacy		
6. Provide Assistive Devices per Care Plan		
7. Adjust bed height to low position. Lock brakes on the bed.		
8. Assist resident to the side of the bed and allow time to gain balance. Put on socks and nonskid shoes.		
9. Put on gait belt around resident's waist. Assist to stand using good body mechanics. Place cane in strong side's hand.		
10. Assist resident to stand by straightening legs as you lift with gait belt as resident pushes down with hands on the mattress.		
11. Instruct resident to move cane forward and a little out to the side of the strong leg.		
12. Instruct resident to move weak extremity forward to line up evenly with tip of cane just after cane is placed.		
13. Instruct resident to put weight on cane and weak foot while swinging strong foot forward, taking a step..		
14. Walk in the same pattern as resident (both move left leg together). Walk distance as prescribed in plan of care or charge nurse direction. Return to bed or chair.		
15. Make the resident comfortable, place signal light within reach, Store lift properly.		
16. Wash hands. Record observations		

The student/employee has satisfactorily completed the procedure and demonstrated competency for the skill: "**Ambulate with Cane**" according to the steps outlined. Ask the student/employee questions about the procedure to assure they understand the process and what the information is used for.

____ ____________

Instructor/Clinical Supervisor Signature Date

Becoming a Certified Nurse Assistant: A Person-Centered Approach

Ambulate with Walker

Competency Sheet-Unit XI, LP 1

Name of Student: ____

Equipment Needed:

Gait Belt	Chair
Walker	

The Student Completed the Following	Yes	No
1. Gather equipment		
2. Identify and greet the resident and introduce yourself		
3. Wash hands		
4. Explain what you are going to do		
5. Provide privacy		
6. Provide Assistive Devices per Care Plan		
7. Adjust bed height to low position. Lock brakes on the bed.		
8. Assist resident to the side of the bed and allow time to gain balance. Put on socks and nonskid shoes.		
9. Put on gait belt around resident's waist. Assist to stand using good body mechanics.		
10. Assist resident to stand by straightening legs as you lift with gait belt as resident pushes down with hands on the mattress. Instruct resident to position body within the frame of the walker.		
11. Instruct resident to move walker forward by lifting it up, moving it forward and setting it down.		
12. Encourage resident to take a step forward with the weak leg and then a step with the strong leg. Encourage the resident to take short steps and keep head up and eyes looking forward.		
13. Ambulate the resident the distance outlined by the charge nurse or plan of care. Remember if the resident loses weight-bearing ability use the emergency procedure for assisting with a fall and don't move the resident until assessed by the charge nurse.		
14. Return resident to bed or chair. To ambulate backward, resident steps back with strong foot, takes a step back with weak foot, then walker is moved back. Assist the resident to feel for arm of chair or top of mattress with his/her hand.		

15. Make the resident comfortable, place signal light within reach, Store lift properly.		
16. Wash hands. Record observations		

The student/employee has satisfactorily completed the procedure and demonstrated competency for the skill: "**Ambulate with Walker**" according to the steps outlined. Ask the student/employee questions about the procedure to assure they understand the process and what the information is used for.

____ ___________

Instructor/Clinical Supervisor Signature Date

Becoming a Certified Nurse Assistant: A Person-Centered Approach

Emergency Transfer Techniques

Competency Sheet: Unit VI, LP 2

Name of Student: ______________________________

Equipment Needed:

Blankets

One-Nurse Blanket Carry (used with a resident smaller than you when you must transport without assistance)

The Student Completed the Following	**Yes**	**No**
1. Fold blanket diagonally with the point downward and the long ends on either side of the resident		
2. Help the resident into a sitting position on the bed.		
3. Wrap the blanket around the resident's back and under the arms like a shawl and then tie the ends of the blanket in a knot. Cross the resident's arms.		
4. Insert your right arm between the knotted blanket (below the knot) and the resident's chest.		
5. Turn your back to the resident, bend your knees, and adjust the blanket comfortably over your right shoulder		
6. Straighten your knees to lift the resident from the bed with a minimum amount of strain or effort. Carry the resident on your back. Support the resident's legs with your left arm.		
7. Carry the resident to Safety.		
Blanket Drag		
1. Unfold the blanket on the floor		
2. Help the resident onto the blanket diagonally		
3. If the resident is wearing shoes, remove them. This eliminates the possibility of the heels catching on stairs or floor obstructions.		
4. Lift the corner of the blanket nearest the resident's head, keeping the resident's off the floor.		
5. Using one or both hands, pull the resident, headfirst, to a place of safety.		
Pack Strap Method		
1. Help the resident to a sitting position.		
2. Grasp the resident's right wrist with your left hand and left wrist with you right hand.		
3. Place your head under the resident's arms (without releasing the wrists) and turn, place your back against the resident's chest so that your shoulders are lower than their armpits.		

4. Pull the resident's arms over your shoulders and across your chest for leverage. Keep resident's wrists firmly grasped.		
5. Lean forward slightly, straighten your knees, and transport the resident to safety.		
Hip Method		
1. Turn the resident on their side, facing you.		
2. Sit on the bed, and place your back against the resident's abdomen		
3. Grasp the resident's knees with one arm and slide your other arm down and across their back.		
4. Stand up slowly while drawing the resident up onto your hips		
5. Carry the resident to safety.		
Cradle Drop (To Blanket)		
1. Unfold the blanket on the floor, facing the side of the bed.		
2. The resident should be in the supine position.		
3. Lift under the resident's knees with one arm and under the shoulders with the other. Guide the resident toward you		
4. Bend on knee and press it against the bed, keeping your foot firmly on the floor.		
5. Lower the resident to the floor by bending your back leg to the floor. Keep your other knee against the bed. Your raised knee will support the resident's knees and legs, and your arms will support their shoulders and head. The cradle formed by your arm and knee will protect their shoulders and head.		
6. Pull the resident toward you and ease them onto the blanket. Drag to safety.		

The student/employee has satisfactorily completed the procedure and demonstrated competency for the skill: "**Emergency Transfer Techniques"** according to the steps outlined. Ask the student/employee questions about the procedure to assure they understand the process and what the information is used for.

______________________________________ ____________

Instructor/Clinical Supervisor Signature Date

Bed to Chair Transfer

Competency Sheet-Unit XI, LP 1

Name of Student: ____________________________

Equipment Needed:

Bed	Chair
Gait Belt	Lap Robe if used

The Student Completed the Following	Yes	No
1. Gather equipment		
2. Identify and greet the resident and introduce yourself		
3. Wash hands		
4. Explain what you are going to do		
5. Provide privacy		
6. Provide Assistive Devices per Care Plan		
7. Adjust bed height to low position. Lock brakes on the bed.		
8. Raise head of bed so that resident is in a sitting position		
9. Assist resident to move over in bed to within 5 or 6" of the edge of the bed.		
10. Assist in putting on socks and nonskid shoes		
11. Position W/C, G/C or Commode on resident's strong side if indicated, if not position as desired.		
12. Place side of chair parallel to the bed. Chair should be touching the bed.		
13. Lock wheels on chair.		
14. If pressure relieving devices are directed in the care plan for the chair assure, they are in place. Raise footrests and remove if possible. If possible, remove the armrest on the side next to the bed.		
15. Position your body facing foot of bed		
16. Assist resident to set on the side of the bed by placing one forearm under resident's shoulders and other behind the knees.		
17. Bend your knees, keep your back straight and stand with feet about 18" apart.		

18. Straighten your hips and knees while shifting weight from front foot to back foot. At the same time, lift resident's head and upper body with one forearm (the one behind the shoulder) and pull the legs (with the arm behind the knees) over the side of the bed.		
19. Apply gait belt.		
20. Allow the resident time to adjust in the sitting position		
21. Stand directly in front of the resident; grasp the back of the belt.		
22. Support the resident's knees and feet with your knees and feet, either knee-to-knee or your knees on the sides of the resident's knees, whatever is comfortable for you and the resident.		
23. Have the resident lean forward while sitting on the edge of the bed.		
24. On the count of three, have the resident push up as much as possible while you pull him/her up by straightening your legs and hips and holding onto the belt.		
25. Pivot your entire body as well as the resident's		
26. Lower the resident into the chair by bending at your knees and hips as the resident sits down.		
27. Adjust footrest and arm rest for resident; cover with lap robe if using.		
28. Place positioning devices for proper body alignment per care plan.		
29. Make the resident comfortable, place signal light within reach,		
30. Wash hands.		

The student/employee has satisfactorily completed the procedure and demonstrated competency for the skill: "**Bed to Chair Transfer**" according to the steps outlined. Ask the student/employee questions about the procedure to assure they understand the process and what the information is used for.

_______________________________________ __________

Instructor/Clinical Supervisor Signature Date

Chair to Bed Transfer (2-Person)

Name of Student: ______________________________

Equipment Needed:

Bed	**Chair**
Gait Belt	

The Student Completed the Following	**Yes**	**No**
1. Gather equipment		
2. Identify and greet the resident and introduce yourself		
3. Wash hands		
4. Explain what you are going to do		
5. Provide privacy		
6. Provide Assistive Devices per Care Plan		
7. Adjust bed height to low position. Lock brakes on the bed.		
8. Raise head of bed and fan fold linens to end of bed.		
9. Position chair at side of bed, facing head of bed		
10. Lock wheels, raise footrests or remove, remove arm rest on the side next to bed if possible		
11. Place or assist resident to place feet on the floor		
12. Remove lap road/blanket if used		
13. Lock wheels on chair.		
14. Apply gait belt		
15. Move resident's buttocks to front are of chair. One nurse assist behind the w/c holds the handles of the w/c and press legs onto wheels to provide stability. One nurse assistant in front stands to one side of w/c with one foot parallel to the side of the wheelchair and one foot at 90 degree to resident's feet in front of the chair.		
16. Nurse Assistant in front bends at the knees and keeping back straight wraps one arm around the resident's back and gently holds area below arm and upper back. Do not pull-on neck or shoulder. Gently tip residents' body toward you. Place other hand on resident's thigh and rock hip toward front of chair. Move to the other side of the chair and		

repeat with the other side. Repeat until resident; s buttocks is positioned at the front edge of the w/c.		
17. CNA at the front: Secure resident by holding upper body and legs and position w/c with armrest parallel and close to the bed. Allow enough room for CNA at the back of the chair to position one foot between w//c and bed.		
18. CNA in front grasp gait belt with palms up. Caution: If resident is unable to assist, both arms should be positioned between CNA's arms to prevent injury to weak extremities.		
19. CNA behind: grasp gait belt, place your knee nearest the bed on bed with foot off the bed. Position other foot on floor between w/c and bed with toes pointed toward front of chair. Grasp gait belt behind resident's back with hand farthest from bed, palm down. With other hand, grasp gait belt at resident's side with palm up.		
20. On the count of three, both CNA's help resident to stand. CNA in back helps by moving from squatting to standing position while keeping back straight and using legs and arms for lifting.		
21. Move the resident over bed. CNA in front: Pivot on balls of feet, being certain not to twist back. CNA behind: guide resident's buttocks over the bed.		
22. Lower resident to sitting position by CNA in front: Bend at your hips and knees. CNA in back: return to squatting position on bed.		
23. Move resident back onto bed further by one CNA in front and the other behind the resident. CNA in front: Grasp bait belt with palms up and position your knees to brace resident's knees. CNA in back: Move behind resident, squat on both knees with feet over opposite side of bed, and grasp gait belt with both palms up. On the count of three position resident's buttock safely on the bed.		
24. Remove gait belt		
25. Assist resident to lying position by placing one arm around shoulders and other under knees. Swing resident's legs onto the bed.		
26. Position resident in center of bed		
27. Cover resident, place positioning devices for proper body alignment per care plan.		
28. Make the resident comfortable, place signal light within reach,		
29. Wash hands.		

The student/employee has satisfactorily completed the procedure and demonstrated competency for the skill: "**Chair to Bed Transfer (2-Person)**" according to the steps outlined. Ask the student/employee questions about the procedure to assure they understand the process and what the information is used for.

____________________________________ ____________

Instructor/Clinical Supervisor Signature Date

Becoming a Certified Nurse Assistant: A Person-Centered Approach

Give ROM Exercises

Competency Sheet-Unit XI, LP 1

Name of Student: ______________________________

Equipment Needed:

The Student Completed the Following	Yes	No
1. Gather equipment		
2. Identify and greet the resident and introduce yourself		
3. Wash hands		
4. Explain what you are going to do		
5. Provide privacy		
6. Provide Assistive Devices per Care Plan		
7. Raise bed to a comfortable working height.		
8. Assist resident to a supine position.		
9. Shoulders: a. Flexion/Extension: i. Support the arm at the wrist and elbow and lift the arm toward the ceiling. Continue lifting the arm over the resident's head until you feel resistance. ii. Slowly lower the arm to the resident's side. b. Abduction/Adduction i. Support the arm at the elbow and shoulder and move the arm out to the side. Continue moving toward the resident's head. ii. Slowly lower the arm to the resident's side. c. Internal/External Rotation i. Move the arm away from the body to shoulder level ii. Bring forward to touch the bed and then backward to touch the bed.		
10. Elbow a. Flexion/Extension i. Bend the arm at the elbow, touch the shoulder, then straighten the arm ii. Bend the arm at the elbow, touch chin, then straighten the arm b. Supination/Pronation i. Hold resident's hand in a handshake position; support the arm at the elbow joint		

ii. Turn plan of hand tard the floor and then toward the ceiling		
11. Wrist a. Flexion/Extension i. Support arm and hand; bend the wrist forward, straighten it, and then bend it backward b. Abduction/Adduction i. Move the hand from side to side at the wrist.		
12. Fingers a. Flexion/Extension i. Support the hand at the wrist. Instruct resident to make a clenched fist and then relax it. Make sure that the thumb is on top of the fingers and open hand fully. b. Abduction/Adduction i. Move each finger away from the nearest finger and then return it. c. Thumb Opposition i. Bend the little finger toward the inner hand and stretch the thumb toward the little finger and move it to the base of the little finger and back. Repeat with each finger. d. Thumb Rotation i. Move the thumb in a circle one direction and then the other direction		
13. Hip and Knee a. Flexion/extension i. Support the leg at the knee and ankle joints and keep the knee straight. Raise and lower the leg. ii. Bend the knee and move toward the chest, slowly straighten the knee. b. Abduction/adduction i. Move the leg straight out to the side of the body until you feel resistance ii. Slowly move the leg back toward the center of the body. c. Internal/external rotation i. Support the knee and ankle joints; move the ankle in toward the opposite leg and then outward.		
14. Ankle a. Inversion/eversion i. Support the foot at the ankle joint and turn the foot toward the opposite foot and then away from the opposite foot. b. Dorsiflexion/plantarflexion i. Bend the foot up toward the knee then down toward the floor.		
15. Toes a. Flexion/extension		

i. Bend and then straighten the toes b. Abduction/adduction i. Move each toe toward the next toe and then away from the next toe.		
16. Make the resident comfortable, place signal light within reach, Store lift properly.		
17. Wash hands. Record observations		

The student/employee has satisfactorily completed the procedure and demonstrated competency for the skill: "**Give ROM Exercises**" according to the steps outlined. Ask the student/employee questions about the procedure to assure they understand the process and what the information is used for.

____ ___________

Instructor/Clinical Supervisor Signature Date

Chair to Bed Transfer

Name of Student: ____

Equipment Needed:

Bed	Chair
Gait Belt	

The Student Completed the Following	Yes	No
1. Gather equipment		
2. Identify and greet the resident and introduce yourself		
3. Wash hands		
4. Explain what you are going to do		
5. Provide privacy		
6. Provide Assistive Devices per Care Plan		
7. Adjust bed height to low position. Lock brakes on the bed.		
8. Raise head of bed and fan fold linens to end of bed.		
9. Position chair at side of bed, facing head of bed		
10. Lock wheels, raise footrests or remove, remove arm rest on the side next to bed if possible		
11. Place or assist resident to place feet on the floor		
12. Remove lap road/blanket if used		
13. Lock wheels on chair.		
14. Apply gait belt		
15. Stand in front of resident with feet about 18" apart		
16. Place your hands underneath belt. If resident is able, have him/her place hands on arms of wheelchair and push. If unable place his/her arms on the CNA arms (not shoulders and necks)		
17. Assist resident to stand (give a few seconds to gain balance).		

18. Pivot your body and the resident's body toward the bed.		
19. Slowly lower resident to sitting position on the bed.		
20. Remove gait belt		
21. Position your body facing the head of the bed. One foot should be in front of the other foot		
22. Place one forearm around resident's shoulders and the other behind the resident's knees		
23. Swing resident's legs onto the bed as you pivot the body.		
24. Lower head of bed		
25. Move/assist resident to center of bed		
26. Lower the resident into the chair by bending at your knees and hips as the resident sits down.		
27. Cover resident, place positioning devices for proper body alignment per care plan.		
28. Make the resident comfortable, place signal light within reach,		
29. Wash hands.		

The student/employee has satisfactorily completed the procedure and demonstrated competency for the skill: "**Chair to Bed Transfer**" according to the steps outlined. Ask the student/employee questions about the procedure to assure they understand the process and what the information is used for.

____________________________________ __________

Instructor/Clinical Supervisor Signature Date

Transfer to Chair with Mechanical Lift (2 person)

Name of Student: ____

Equipment Needed:

Bed	Chair
Mechanical Lift	

The Student Completed the Following	Yes	No
1. Gather equipment		
2. Identify and greet the resident and introduce yourself		
3. Wash hands		
4. Explain what you are going to do		
5. Provide privacy		
6. Provide Assistive Devices per Care Plan		
7. Adjust bed height to low position. Lock brakes on the bed.		
8. Position chair at side of bed, with back of chair in line with the headboard of the bed.		
9. Turn resident from side to side to position the lift sling under the resident with the top of the sling at the crest of the shoulders and the bottom above the bend of the knees.		
10. Wheel the lift into place over the resident with the base beneath the bed and be sure to lock the wheels of the lift. Widen the base of the lift.		
11. Open support legs of the lift with the control lever. Never close legs while transporting residents.		
12. Attach sling to mechanical lift with hooks in place under the metal frame. Assure sharp end of hooks are pointed away from resident.		
13. Using crank, lift resident until buttocks are clear of bed. Assure resident alignment in the sling and is securely suspended in a sitting position with legs dangling over the bottom of the sling.		
14. One CNA guides the resident's legs over the edge of the bed; release the breaks on the lift.		

15. Move lift away from bed, turn the resident so that they face you while the other CNA guides the resident's body toward the chair by standing behind the resident.		
16. Bring lift into position so that the resident is over the seat of the chair. Lower the resident to the chair while the second CNA guides the hips into proper alignment in the chair.		
17. Remove hooks from the lift frame and pull lift away. If sling is left in place assure it is flat and not wrinkled up under resident otherwise remove it.		
18. Make the resident comfortable, place signal light within reach, Store lift properly.		
19. Wash hands.		

The student/employee has satisfactorily completed the procedure and demonstrated competency for the skill: "**Transfer to Chair with Mechanical Lift (2 person)**" according to the steps outlined. Ask the student/employee questions about the procedure to assure they understand the process and what the information is used for.

_______________________________________ ___________

Instructor/Clinical Supervisor Signature Date

Becoming a Certified Nurse Assistant: A Person-Centered Approach

Move Resident to the Head of Bed (2-Person Assist)

Name of Student: ______________________________

Equipment Needed:

Lift Sheet	

The Student Completed the Following	Yes	No
1. Gather equipment		
2. Identify and greet the resident and introduce yourself		
3. Wash hands		
4. Explain what you are going to do		
5. Provide privacy		
6. Provide Assistive Devices per Care Plan		
7. Raise bed to a comfortable working height, lock wheels on bed. Lower the head of bed; lower side rail if applicable		
8. Assure that any tubing (catheters, g-tubes) are free from any anchor points (pinned to sheets, etc.)		
9. Move the pillow so that it rests against the headboard of the bed to prevent damage to the resident's head if bumped against the headboard.		
10. CNA's stand on opposite sides of the bed of each other (one on either side of the resident)		
11. Position a lift sheet/folded regular sheet under shoulders and hip area. CNA should roll edges of sheet toward resident's body and grasp rolled sheet with his/her hands (with palms up) at the resident's shoulders and at the mid-hip area.		
12. Point your feet in the direction you are moving the resident; bend knees, keep back straight		
13. On the count of three, each CNA lifts the resident with the rolled sheet. Lift off the surface of the bed and toward the head of the bed while shifting the CNA's weight from the back foot to the front foot.		
14. Replace Pillow under the resident's head and adjust back rest to the comfort of the resident. Lower the bed to a position of safety.		
15. Assure the resident's comfort and that the call signal is within reach. Refasten any tubing that you loosened to move the resident.		
16. Wash hands.		

The student/employee has satisfactorily completed the procedure and demonstrated competency for the skill: "**Move Resident to the Head of Bed (2-Person Assist)**" according to the steps outlined. Ask the student/employee questions about the procedure to assure they understand the process and what the information is used for.

____ ___________

Instructor/Clinical Supervisor Signature Date

Becoming a Certified Nurse Assistant: A Person-Centered Approach

Turn Resident to Side (Lateral Position)

Name of Student: ______________________________________

Equipment Needed:

Three pillows-additional blankets/washcloths as needed	Handroll/washcloth

The Student Completed the Following	Yes	No
1. Gather equipment		
2. Identify and greet the resident and introduce yourself		
3. Wash hands		
4. Explain what you are going to do		
5. Provide privacy		
6. Provide Assistive Devices per Care Plan		
7. Raise bed to a comfortable working height, lock wheels on bed. Lower the head of bed; lower side rail if applicable		
8. Assure that any tubing (catheters, g-tubes) are free from any anchor points (pinned to sheets, etc.)		
9. Loosen the top sheets without exposing the resident. Remove pillow.		
10. Cross the resident's arms over his/her chest		
11. Cross the leg farthest from you over the leg closest to you.		
12. Reach across the resident and put one hand behind his/her far shoulder		
13. Place your other hand behind his/her far hip and gently roll him/her toward you.		
14. Fold a pillow lengthwise and place it against the resident's back for support. As you face the resident, pull the side of the lift sheet that is closest to you slightly toward you.		
15. Support the resident's head with the palm of one hand and slide a pillow under his/her head and neck with the other hand.		
16. Position resident's knees slightly flexed, upper leg more than the lower leg. Support upper leg on pillow		
17. Support upper arm on pillow.		
18. Rotate lower shoulder slightly toward you so that pressure is not on the bone.		

19. Place hand roll or rolled washcloth in clean, dry hand with thumb in opposition to fingers and according to care plan,		
20. Make the resident comfortable, place signal light within reach, fasten any tubing that was loosened, and adjust the bedding.		
21. Lower bed to a position of safety		
22. Wash hands.		

The student/employee has satisfactorily completed the procedure and demonstrated competency for the skill: "**Turn Resident to Side (Lateral Position)**" according to the steps outlined. Ask the student/employee questions about the procedure to assure they understand the process and what the information is used for.

______________________________________ __________

Instructor/Clinical Supervisor Signature Date

Becoming a Certified Nurse Assistant: A Person-Centered Approach

Measure Weight and Height

Competency Sheet: Unit III, LP 4

Name of Student: ________________________________

Equipment Needed:

Scale (upright or platform)
Chart or form for recording
Pen and Paper

The Student Completed the Following	Yes	No
1. Gathered the necessary equipment		
2. Identify and greet the resident. Identify Self		
3. Wash your hands. Glove if needed.		
4. Wash your hands. Glove if needed.		
5. Provide privacy.		
6. Raise the measuring rod on the upright scale.		
7. Ask resident to remove robe, slippers aid as needed.		
8. Ask the resident to stand on the scale platform; have them stand with arms to the side.		
9. Read the weight. When using a balance scale, move the weight until the pointer swings evenly between the top and bottom of the metal square. This is usually the weight.		
10. Record weight. Review last recorded weight if more than 2# variance reweigh.		
11. Instruct the resident to stand upright.		
12. Lower the measuring rod until it rests on the resident's head.		
13. Read the height and record it on paper. Raise measuring rod to remove it from the resident's head.		
14. Assist resident off the scale and putting back robe and slippers. Assist to bed or chair.		
15. . Wash hands.		
16. Make resident comfortable and place call signal within reach.		
17. Remove, clean and store equipment.		
18. Record observations and report anything unusual to the charge nurse.		

Becoming a Certified Nurse Assistant: A Person-Centered Approach

The student/employee has satisfactorily completed the procedure and demonstrated competency for the skill: "**Measure Weight and Height**" according to the steps outlined. Ask the student/employee questions about the procedure to assure they understand the process and what the information is used for.

____ _______________

Instructor/Clinical Supervisor Signature Date

Becoming a Certified Nurse Assistant: A Person-Centered Approach

Emergency First Aid for Chemical Exposures

Competency Sheet: Unit VI, LP 1

Name of Student: ____

Equipment Needed:
Material Safety Data Sheets or Safety Data Sheets
Poison Control Emergency Number
Water As Needed for Flushing Skin Exposure

The Student Completed the Following	Yes	No
1. If you suspect that a resident has been exposed such as breathing, splashing on skin or inhaling or ingesting (swallowing) a potentially hazardous chemical		
2. Follow the guidelines in the MSDS sheet for the chemical. Call for help from the charge nurse and follow his/her instructions.		
3. Locate the Poison Control Centers Helpline		
4. If the resident inhaled the chemical get them to fresh air as quickly as possible.		
5. If the splashed the chemical on their skin, rinse it off with lots of running water.		
6. If they ingested (swallowed) it, **do not** induce vomiting. Rinse the mouth out.		
7. Follow poison control centers' guidance and the first aid response on the MSDS sheet		
8. If the chemical splashed in the eyes, flush with cool running water for at least 5 minutes. Remove contact lens if appliable. Then continue flushing for at least 15 minutes holding the eyelids open to ensure the entire eye is rinsed.		
9. Assist the resident back to a bed or a chair and follow the charge nurse's instruction for further observations post incident (such as transport to emergency room).		
10. Assist with the Incident report as requested		
11. Wash hands.		
12. Make resident comfortable and place call signal within reach if not transferred to ER.		
13. Record observations and report anything unusual to the charge nurse.		

The student/employee has satisfactorily completed the procedure and demonstrated competency for the skill: "**Emergency First Aid for Chemical Exposure"** according to the steps outlined. Ask the student/employee questions about the procedure to assure they understand the process and what the information is used for.

____ ____________

Instructor/Clinical Supervisor Signature Date

Becoming a Certified Nurse Assistant: A Person-Centered Approach

Emergency First Aid for Electrical Burns

Competency Sheet: Unit VI, LP 1

Name of Student: ______________________________

The Student Completed the Following	Yes	No
1. Turn off the source of electricity if possible. If not call 911 and seek help disabling electrical current (maintenance). Do not touch the person if they are still being shocked by the electrical source,		
2. Begin CPR if the person shows no signs of circulation, such as breathing, coughing or movement.		
3. Call for help and await the charge nurse.		
4. Assist the charge nurse to apply a bandage. Cover any burned areas with a sterile gauze bandage, if available, or a clean cloth. Don't use a blanket or towel, because loose fibers can stick to the burns.		
5. For mild skin burn cool the burn by putting a cool cloth on the burn or soaking it in cool water, Do not put ice on the burn.		
6. Visible electrical burns can indicate underlying tissue damage and will likely require evaluation at the ER.		
7. Assist the resident back to a bed or a chair and follow the charge nurse's instruction for further observations post incident (such as transport to emergency room).		
8. Assist with the Incident report as requested		
9. Wash hands.		
10. Make resident comfortable and place call signal within reach if not transferred to ER.		
11. Record observations and report anything unusual to the charge nurse.		

The student/employee has satisfactorily completed the procedure and demonstrated competency for the skill: "**Emergency First Aid for Electrical Burns"** according to the steps outlined. Ask the student/employee questions about the procedure to assure they understand the process and what the information is used for.

______________________________ __________

Instructor/Clinical Supervisor Signature Date

Becoming a Certified Nurse Assistant: A Person-Centered Approach

Administer Oxygen by Nasal Cannula

Unit XII, LP 1

Name of Student: ____

Equipment Needed:

No Smoking Signs	Nasal Cannula Tubing
Humidification Container	**Flow meter if not already on the device**
Distilled Water	

The Student Completed the Following	Yes	No
1. Gather equipment		
2. Identify and greet the resident and introduce yourself		
3. Wash hands- and put-on gloves		
4. Explain what you are going to do		
5. Provide privacy		
6. Post No Smoking signs per facility policy		
7. If resident is to have humidifier bottle fill to 2/3rd with distilled water and attach to oxygen flow meter.		
8. Attach the connecting tube from the nasal cannula to the humidifier		
9. The nurse should set the flow meter at the prescribed amount of oxygen		
10. Assist the nurse to place the tips of the cannula in the person's nose and adjust straps around ears for a snug, comfortable fit		
11. Wash resident's hands and then wash your own.		
12. Make resident comfortable and assure call light is in reach		
13. Record observations and report anything unusual to charge nurse		

The student/employee has satisfactorily completed the procedure and demonstrated competency for the skill: "**Administer Oxygen with Nasal Cannula"** according to the steps outlined. Ask the student/employee questions about the procedure to assure they understand the process and what the information is used for.

____ ____________

Instructor/Clinical Supervisor Signature Date

Becoming a Certified Nurse Assistant: A Person-Centered Approach

Administer Oxygen by Simple Face Mask

Unit XII, LP 1

Name of Student: ____

Equipment Needed:

No Smoking Signs	Face Mask and Tubing per orders
Humidification Container	
Distilled Water	

The Student Completed the Following		Yes
1. Gather equipment		
2. Identify and greet the resident and introduce yourself		
3. Wash hands- and put-on gloves		
4. Explain what you are going to do		
5. Provide privacy		
6. Post No Smoking signs per facility policy		
7. If resident is to have humidifier bottle fill to 2/3rd with distilled water and attach to oxygen flow meter.		
8. Attach the connecting tube from the nasal cannula to the humidifier		
9. The nurse should set the flow meter at the prescribed amount of oxygen		
10. Assist the nurse to place the face mask on the person's face and adjusting straps so the mask fits securely. If tubing fills with water drain through mask do not drain back into the humidified water container. If heating element is used check the temperature. The humidifier bottle should feel warm, not hot, to touch.		
11. Wash resident's hands and then wash your own.		
12. Make resident comfortable and assure call light is in reach		
13. Record observations and report anything unusual to charge nurse		

The student/employee has satisfactorily completed the procedure and demonstrated competency for the skill: "**Administer Oxygen with Simple Face Mask**" according to the steps outlined. Ask the student/employee questions about the procedure to assure they understand the process and what the information is used for.

____ ______________

Instructor/Clinical Supervisor Signature Date

Assist with Incentive Spirometer

Unit XII, LP 1

Name of Student: ____

Equipment Needed:

Pillow for splinting (if needed)	Note: IF resident has had surgery this should be done approximately 30 minutes after the administration of pain medication. Coordinate with the nurse.
Incentive Spirometer	Alcohol Wipes

The Student Completed the Following	Yes	No
1. Gather equipment		
2. Identify and greet the resident and introduce yourself		
3. Wash hands- and put-on gloves		
4. Explain what you are going to do		
5. Provide privacy		
6. Assist the person to a comfortable sitting or semi-fowlers position. If recent surgery uses the pillow to splint the incision site. (on top of incision site-resident may hold pressure against it)		
7. Set the spirometer according to the instructions provided by the charge nurse or as noted in the orders or care plan.		
8. Instruct the person to exhale fully, place the mouthpiece into the mouth, and keep lips sealed tightly around the mouthpiece.		
9. Direct the resident to inhale (breathe in) slowly and deeply, trying to reach the goal by watching the ball move up in the spirometer tube to the level set.		
10. When the goal is met or the ball will move no further instruct the person to hold the breath for three seconds, remove the mouthpiece, relax ad exhale (breathe out). Encourage the person to cough and praise their results.		
11. Wash resident's hands and then wash your own.		
12. Make resident comfortable and assure call light is in reach		
13. Record observations and report anything unusual to charge nurse or inability to meet goals.		

The student/employee has satisfactorily completed the procedure and demonstrated competency for the skill: "**Assist with Incentive Spirometer"** according to the steps outlined. Ask the student/employee questions about the procedure to assure they understand the process and what the information is used for.

____ ___________

Instructor/Clinical Supervisor Signature Date

Give Postmortem Care

Name of Student: ________________________________

Equipment Needed:

Wash Cloth	
Towel	**Clean Gown**
Bath Basin	
Resident's Comb	**Gloves**
Clean Linen	

The Student Completed the Following	Yes	No
1. Gather equipment		
2. Ask charge nurse to remove tubing, catheters, or IV's and to change dressings. Take jewelry and belongings to charge nurse.		
3. Wash hands- and put-on gloves		
4. Flatten bed and straighten the body		
5. Provide privacy		
6. Elevate the head of the bed slightly or put a pillow under the head and neck.		
7. Close eyes by gently holding in place a few moments		
8. Place dentures in cup per facility policy and assure they are transported with the resident.		
9. Give a bed bath		
10. Comb hair		
11. Place a clean gown on resident		
12. Wipe lips with a towel		
13. Arrange linen neatly		
14. Straighten room and remove, clean and store equipment		
15. Remove gloves and dispose of appropriately		
16. Provide Privacy for the Family		

Becoming a Certified Nurse Assistant: A Person-Centered Approach

The student/employee has satisfactorily completed the procedure and demonstrated competency for the skill: "**Administer Postmortem Care"** according to the steps outlined. Ask the student/employee questions about the procedure to assure they understand the process and what the information is used for.

____ ___________

Instructor/Clinical Supervisor Signature Date

NURSE AIDE TRAINING PROGRAM EVALUATION

Please complete this evaluation after you have completed the Nurse Aide Training Program:

Did you feel that the number of hours of classroom time were adequate for your learning needs?

YES or NO

Did you feel the number of hours of On-The-Job Training were adequate for your learning needs?

YES or NO

Did the instructor portray a professional mannerism?

YES or NO

Was the instructor knowledgeable on nurse aide training?

YES or NO

What was the name of your primary nurse aide training instructor? ____

Did you have any other instructors for your nurse aide training?

____

Are you comfortable taking care of residents or patients in the healthcare setting in which you will be working?

YES or NO

Did you feel you were adequately supervised by the instructor or clinical supervisor during your classroom or on-the-job training?

YES or NO

Was the instructor/clinical supervisor readily available to answer questions, demonstrate procedures, and support your training experience?

YES or NO

Was there time allowed for questions to be answered?

YES or NO

Do you feel you received a quality education?

YES or NO

Would you recommend this Nurse Aide Training Program to a friend?

YES or NO

Did you ever feel that you were being asked to do any procedure or offer any care that you had not been adequately trained in or that you were asked to do something before you were ready?

YES or NO

What did you enjoy the most in the classroom experience?

What did you not enjoy about the classroom experience if anything?

What did you enjoy the most about the On-the-job training experience?

What did you not enjoy about the On-the-job training experience, if anything?

CPSIA information can be obtained
at www.ICGtesting.com
Printed in the USA
LVHW060021080323
741158LV00024B/182

9 781716 348679